Healing Touch

Ayurvedic Massage

THE
CHAUKHAMBA AYURVIJNAN STUDIES
30

Healing Touch

Ayurvedic Massage

BY

Prof. Subhash Ranade
B.A.M.& S.; M.A.Sc, Ph.D.

Dr. Rajan Rawat
B.A.M. S., D.N.T.Y.M.

CHAUKHAMBHA SANSKRIT PRATISHTHAN
DELHI

First Edition : Delhi, 2000
© Authors
ISBN : 81-7084-149-6

Published by
CHAUKHAMBA SANSKRIT PRATISHTHAN
38 U.A., Bungalow Road, Jawahar Nagar,
Post Box N0. 2113
Delhi 110007

Also available at
CHOWKHAMBA VIDYABHAWAN
Chowk, Post Box No. 1069
Varanasi 221001

CHAUKHAMBA SURBHARATI PRAKASHAN
K 37/117, Gopal Mandir Lane,
Post Box N0. 1129
Varanasi 221001

Printed by
A. K. Lithographers

Preface

Massage is an ancient Indian art used for healing, relaxation as well as for treating various diseases. Touch can bring about dramatic changes in body and mind. Ayurvedic massage has many advantages over any other oriental or modern systems of massage.

Ayurvedic massage is done according to constitution, age, stage of the disease, aggravated doshas, status of agni and ama. With this subtle understanding Ayurvedic masseur can choose correct type of oil or other substances for massage, that can bring dramatic results for healthy as well as for diseased perosn.

Inspite of development of sophisticated equipment for treating various physical injuries and wide range of electrical apperatus it is quite surprising that after understanding fundamental principles of Ayurveda, if correct oil or other substances and methods are used, they givemuch better results.

Many authors have written about Ayurvedic massage. However very few have given proper consideration to the basic principles of Ayurveda. Therefore while writing this book we have explained all fundamental principles of Ayurveda in the first five chapters. Later on we have explained various methods as well as oils and other substances used for masage.

For the first time, we have explained very important concept of 'Marma massage' which is becoming very popular not only in India but Abroad also.

The chapter on 'Massage for specific Diseases' will no doubt attract attention of the readers, as it has highlighted some important diseases in which massage can be very useful. We have given more than 90 illustrations for explaining various basic principles and methods of massage. This addition will make the book more readable and useful to the people.
We hope that this book will receive good response from Ayurvedic as well as other scientific community.

Authors are thankful to Dr. Hans H. Rhyner, Dr. Prasanna Paranjape, and Dr. Ajit Mandalecha and for providing valuable material and helpful suggestions.

Prof. Subhash Ranade
Rajbharati, 367 Sahakar Nagar 1
Pune, India. 411,009
E Mail- sbranade@hotmail.com

Dr. Rajan Rawat
'Shri' 38,Shamsundar
Hsg.Soc., Pune,
India, 411,030

Illustrations

Contents

◆ ◆◆◆ ◆

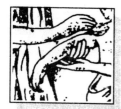

1.
History of Massage

Massage is perhaps the most popular form of health activity today. It is effectively used for achieving relaxation and as a form of natural therapy for various diseases also. The art of massage has been practiced since ancient times and in many countries.

A word for massage exists in all cultures we have known and from studies of the classics, it would appear that ancient Chinese, Greeks, and Romans all practiced a form of massage. Roman and Greek philosophers and physicians prescribed massage both for its restorative powers after battel and for general health of body and mind. Ancient Greeks had set up massage schools in their gymnasiums. They were using massage for maintaining health as well as for treating various diseases.

The famous literature of odyssey by Homer mentions, that beautiful girls gave massage to the fatigued soldiers who returned from the war. In the Far East, performing musicians and actors learned massage practices to aid their artistic development. The same is true in Kerala - south India, where massage after *Kathakali* dance is given to all the artists for reducing the fatigue. Similarly, Indian cultures and their epics like *Ramayana* and *Mahabharata* have described massage for health maintenance.

Bhavishya Purna, which is also very old text, has mentioned different techniques of massage. This also mentions how wife should give massage to her husband. Importance of pressure on different organs has also been described during the massage

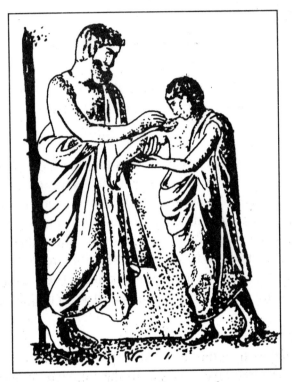

Ancient Massage inRoman culture

procedures e.g. light pressure should be given on face, neck while more pressure can be given on thighs and back region. Usually the massage should be done in the direction of hairs.

Similarly in *Vatsyayana Kamasutra*, massage has been explained for the purpose of enhancing the sexual power. This text has mentioned three different types - *samvahana* (whole body massage), *keshamardana* (head massage) and *utsadana* (massage done by feet). The text has described the art of massage as one of the 64 *Kalas* (arts).

Marma Massage - Massage to vital points on the body called as *'marma,'* is the specialty of Ayurveda. The origin can be traced to *Saraswati* Culture or Indus Valley Civilization. It is known from various excavations at *Harrappa* and *Mohen-jo -daro* that people in this culture were using various types of weapons in war and to protect from the injuries they were using the knowledge of these vital points.

In Vedic period also people were using different weapons like axes, spears, daggers, maces, bows and arrows. These were made of copper or bronze. For defensive purpose they were using body shields. Knowledge of Marma exists from very ancient time of Vedas, which dates back 4000 BC. The first reference is found in Rig-Veda. There is reference of words like *Varman* and *drapi,* which is some kind of body armor or corselet to protect the body from the assault of enemy weapons. In *Atharva-Veda* also we find the reference of the term *kavacha* or corselet or breastplate for the protection. In *Mahabharata* the great epic also we find many references for *marma* or *varman*. (*Karnaparva* 19.31, *Shalyaparva* 32.63 and 36.64, *Dronaparva* 125.17, *Bhishmaparva* 95.47, *Virataparva* 31.12 and 15). It is interesting that there are references of protective clothing of the marmas of elephants and horses also. *Arhashastra* of *Kautilya* mentions the use of arrowheads made up of metal and some protective instruments against the injury to marmas.

Later on during the period of Buddha, this art spread in the

3

neighboring countries like Indonesia, Burma, Tibet and China. In some societies massage has been used socially as an act of hospitality as in Hawaii. Passive movements called Lomi-Lomi are bestowed on honored guests. Early physicians were able to use massage effectively in treating fatigue, illness and injury.

Along with *'bruhat trayi'* the technique of massage has been explained in detail in texts like *yogratnakara*, *bhavaprakasha* etc.

In 18 th century massage was regularly given to the sportsmen as well as to the soldiers. Massage became very popular in Euorpe due to the work of Per Henrik Ling. He was sweedish and after visiting China he set up his own method of massage, which later on became very popular throughtout the World. Later on in 19 th century, two separate branches physiotherapy and occupational therapy came into existence.

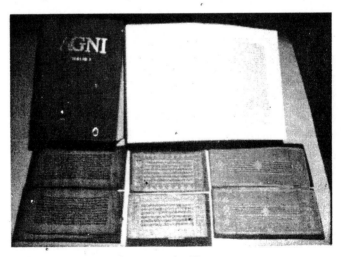

Ayurvedic Text

4

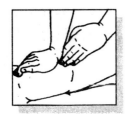

2.
Basic Principles of Ayurveda

Ayurveda is one of the great gifts of the sages of ancient India to mankind. It is one of the oldest scientific medical systems in the world with a long record of clinical experience to validate it. However, it is not only a system of medicine in the conventional sense of curing disease. It is also a way of life that teaches us how to maintain and protect health. It shows us how to both cure disease and to promote longevity. Ayurveda treats man as a 'whole'- though at the same time viewing him as a combination of body, mind, and soul. Therefore it is a truly holistic and integral medical system.

The word *'Ayu,'* means all aspects of life from birth to death. The word 'Veda' means knowledge or learning. Thus *'Ayurveda'* denotes the science by which life in its totality is understood. It is a science of life that delineates the diet, medicines, and behavior that are beneficial or harmful for life.

Ayurveda originated in the very beginning of the cosmic creation. Indian philosophers state that Ayurveda originates from *Brahma*, the creator of the universe. *Brahma* is not a mere individual but the unmanifest form of the Divine Lord, from whom the whole manifest world has come into being. The desire to keep fit, healthy, and live long is found in the basic instincts of each organism. In this respect Ayurveda is the paradigm for other systems of medicine. Hence Ayurveda is a tradition with an antiquity concurrent with that of life itself.

Ayurveda accepts the concept of a common origin of the universe and man. The universe is the macrocosm, while man is the microcosm. For the creation of the universe two types of substances are essential: material and non-material.

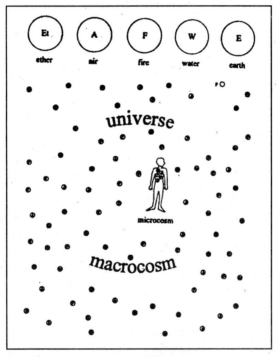

Macrocosm - Microcosm

Trigunas - **Super qualities**

Sattva, consciousness or knowledge, *Rajas*, motion or action, and *Tamas*, inertia resisting them is called the three *gunas* (*trigunas*). They are the three ultimate qualities at work in nature behind all material forms. For the creation of any

6

substance in the universe the contribution of these three non-material substances is essential.

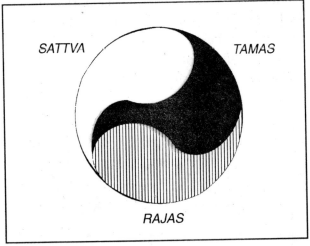

Triguna

Quantum physics - *Panchamahabhootas*
The basic material constituents who exist in the universe and in man are called the five great elements, *Pancha Mahabhutas*. They are ether (*akasha*), air (*vayu*), fire (*tejas*), water (*apa*) and earth (*prithvi*). The origin and substratum of this group, which itself is not completely observable, pervades the universe and is known as *Mahabhutas*, the Great Element.

Ether - space, Air - Motion, Fire - Energy, heat, Water - Liquid, Earth - Solid mass are the principles of density that applies to all manifest mediums, including mind. Earth on one hand is completely dense medium that allows no action and Ether on the other hand is completely subtle and receptive medium that allows complete freedom. Between these two polarities are all possible densities.

7

As long as all these primordial elements in Universe are in equilibrium, all the Universal activities are in proper order. Once these elements are imbalanced, natural calamities occur like floods, cyclones, earthquakes, and extremes of heat and cold. In the human being also these elements must remain in proper balance, then only the health of the individual is maintained. Due to their imbalance, all types of disorders can take place in man.

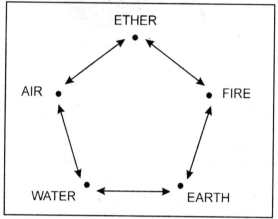

Primordial Elements

Due to excess element of ether, deformities like osteoporosis, cavities in lungs can take place. When solid tumors and hypertrophy of organs takes place, ether element gets decreased. Due to excess element of air, deformities like tremors, tachycardia occurs in the body, while due to its decrease, paresis and paralysis and improper movement of muscles can take place in the body. Due to excess element of fire in the body, all types of inflammations, fever, ulcers can occur, while due to its decrease, deformities like hyper-pigmentation, anemia take place.

Due to excess accumulation of water in the body, deformities like edema, pleurisy, ascites can take place, while because of its decrease dehydration takes place. Due to excess element of earth, different solid tumors of bones and obesity can occur, while due to its decrease there are deformities like loss of weight can take place.

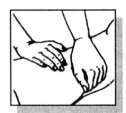

3.
Ayurvedic Anatomy

Description of Organs

Various texts have described in detail the number and descriptions of the bones, muscles, tendons, nerves, veins, and arteries. Since at that time the method of dissecting dead bodies was different from that of today, the description and the numbers of these organs may differ from modern textbooks of anatomy. But, more importantly, their function in relation to each other is very accurate.

Sushruta has explained various organs and their numbers in detail -

1. Bones (*asthi*) - 300 (Modern anatomy has described 206 bones, while in Ayurveda all the cartilage's have been included in bones.); Extremities - 120, Trunk and chest- 117 Head and Neck - 63.

Our bones are known collectively as skeleton, which means 'dried up'. Contrary to their appearance after death, they are extremely dynamic and versatile structures, which protect major important organs and give support and strength to the body.

2. Joints (*sandhi*) - 210; Extremities- 68, Trunk-59, Head and Neck- 83.

    The bony joints have been divided in three types -

    i) Movable - Hinge joints (*kora*) - knee, (*Ulukhala*) and ball and socket joint (hip, shoulder).

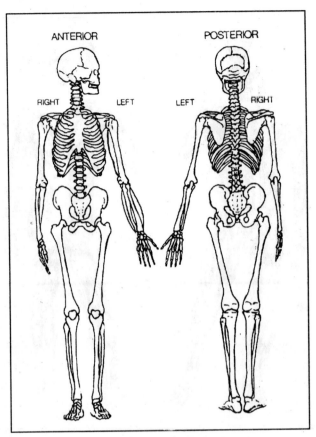

Bony Skeleton

 ii) Partially movable - Saddle joint (*samugda*)-sacro-iliac or clavicle, (*Pratara*) - joint in between vertebras and (*vayastunda*)- like beak of crow-tempero -mandibular.

 iii) Non-movable - (*Tunna sevani*)- Joints in skull bones.

3. Ligaments (*snayu*)- 900; Extremities - 600, Trunk -230, Head and Neck -70

4. Muscles (*peshi*)- 500; Extremities- 400, Trunk- 66, Head and Neck-34

When muscle tissue forms different shapes due to the action

11

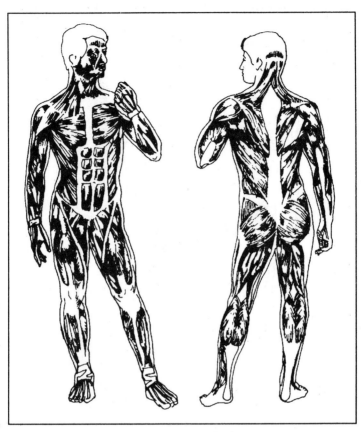

Muscles in the body

of *Vata*, it is called as *Peshi*.

There are 12 types of *peshi* in the body -
Bahala - large muscles like biceps and triceps.
Pelava - very small - around metacarpal or metatarsal bones of hand and feet. They originate from the carpal tunnels.
Sthoola - very big- like muscles on the buttocks- gluteus major.
Anu - extremely small - like muscles in the eyeball.
Pruthu - big flat muscles on chest- pectoralis major.

Vrutta - round shape- muscles over the shoulder joint- deltoid.

Kathina - hard muscles on thigh- quadriceps.

Mrudu - soft - around eye - orbicularis oculi.

Deergha - long - muscles from shoulder joint to the arm-pronator longus.

Rooksha - rough - in large intestines.

Hrasva - short - muscles in wrist joint.

Muscles are every where in our body, making up the mass of our weight and shape. Muscles record our feelings and their tensions help ease stressful situations. However, when this tension is not relaxed sufficienlty, the lining of the muscles and the surrounding tissues get irritated, creating fibrositis.

5. Tendons (*kandara*) - 16; Extremities-8, Trunk-4, Head and Neck-4

6. Vessels (*Sira*) - 700; This includes veins and arteries.

Skin

Skin is very important structure for massage. It is related with various doshas, sub-doshas, *srotasas* or channels.

In 'ancient period of *Sushruta* and *Charaka* although instruments like microscope were not available, both these authors have described 7 and 6 layers of the skin respectively and the diseases that originate from each of these layers.

Sushruta has given names to all the 7 layers while *Charaka* has given names only to the first 2 layers.

1. *Avabhasini* - This first layer is connected with *rasa* or plasma. *Charaka* has named this as *Udakadhara*. (This can be compared with stratum cornium). *Sidhma kushtha* a type of skin disease originates from this layer.

2. *Lohita - Asrugdhara* - This second layer is the seat of *rakta* or blood vessels (Stratum lucidium). Moles are in this layer.

3. *Shweta* - This third layer is the place of mamsa or muscles.

13

This layer is the seat of *charmadala* - type of skin disease. (Stratum granulosum).

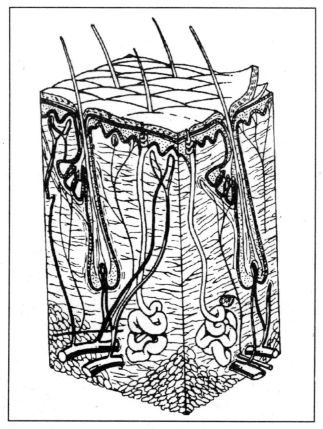

Structure of the skin

4. *Tamra* - This is the forth layer and is the seat of *meda* or fatty tissue, which is connected with diseases like erysipelas or vitiligo. (Stratum spinosum).
5. *Vedini* - This fifth layer is seat of nerve endings (Stratum basale).
6. *Rohini* - Sixth layer is connected with deeper blood vessels and lymph vessels (Papillary and reticular region).

7. *Mamsadhara* - The seventh layer is the seat of sweat glands and all types of abscesses, fistula etc. take place in this layer only. (Subcutaneous layer).

Skin is related with channels of water metabolism, plasma, blood, fatty tissue and the muscular tissue along with nervous tissue. Although it is connected with all the *tridosha*, one can say that *Prana-Vyana* types of *Vata; Bhrajaka Pitta* and *Kledaka Kapha* are closely related with the skin.

Different oils that are applied for the purpose of massage and various ointments are absorbed from the skin because of the action of *Bhrajaka Pitta* along with *Vata Dosha*. Gentle and soothing touch to the skin is also responsible for calming the nerves and mind and can produce excellent relaxing effect.

Marmas -Vital points

Marma points are important pressure points on the body, much like the acupuncture points of traditional Chinese Medicine. The first reference to them is found in the *Atharva Veda*, and *Sushruta* elaborately deals them with. (There is also a reference of '*Suchi-Veda*' which is the origin of acupuncture.) Knowledge of these 107 sensitive anatomical points was applied in war for harming the enemy or protecting oneself. This knowledge became an essential part of the training for surgeons, as injury to these points can produce death or disability.

Definition of marma
1. Marma point is defined as anatomical site where muscle, veins, ligaments, bones and joints meet together. (*Mamsa, sira, snayu, asthi and sandhi* - Su.sh.6/2). This does not mean that all the structures must be present collectively at

15

the site of marma.

2. According to *Ashtang hridaya* these are the points where important nerves (*Dhamani*) come together along with other structures like muscles, tendons etc. *Vagbhata* says that those sites which are painful, severe tender and show abnormal pulsation (should also be) considered as marma or vital points (A.H. sh. 4/ 37). These points are the seats of 'life.' (A.H. sh. 4/ 2) They are also the sites where not only *tridosha* (*Vata, Pitta and Kapha*) are present but their subtle forms *Prana, Ojus (soma)* and *Tejas (agni)* are also

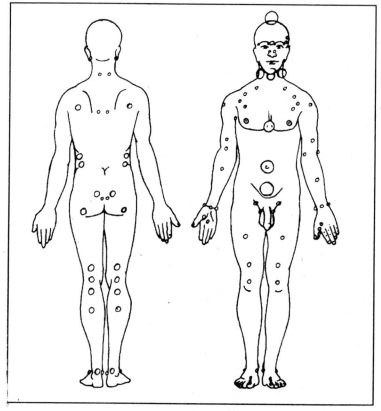

Marma Points

16

present with *sattva*, *rajas* and *tamas* - (Su. sh. 6 / 22, 45). Hence this is a specific area on the body, which has relation through Pranic channel to various internal organs.

4. According to another definition, they are '*Marayanti iti Marmani*' (Dalhan) meaning these are the vital areas, (some of them if injured) which can produce death. If marmas are injured they do not always result into death but can cause various diseases, which are difficult to cure. (*Uttara Rama Charita*). This naturally indicates that all vital points do not produce death when injured.

5. Marma or the vital points on the body, are the junction of the body and mind. They are also important pressure points on the body much like the acupuncture points of the Traditional Chinese Medicine.

The most important difference between acupuncture points and *marma* is the size. The *marma* points are measured in *anguli* or finger unit relative to each individual, and they are larger in size. Also these points are not related to meridians.

<u>Composition of *Marma*</u>

1. *Mamsa* - various structures like facia, serous membranes and sheaths can be compared with *mamsa*. *Sushruta* has stated that *Vata dosha* divides *peshi* and forms muscle.

2. *Sira* - These are like channels supplying water or energy to the field or body. *Sushruta* has explained 4 types of *sira*. Various experts have tried to correlate these structures with some modern anatomical structures. However the explanation is not satisfactory. Still it is certain that these are channels - *srotas*- channels - which carry vital fluids or energy to the entire body.

3. *Snayu* - These are the sub tissues which bind the bones and muscles (Su. sh. 5/42). They are of 4 types - ligaments,

tendons, sphincter muscles and apponurosis.
4. *Asthi* - These can be classified into - bones proper, cartilages, teeth and nails.
5. *Sandhi* - The bony joints are again classified into - movable, partially movable and non-movable.

1. According to the structure

Structure	A.*Hridaya*	A.*Sangraha*	*Sushruta*
Mamsa	10	11	11
Sira	37	41	41
Snayu	23	27	27
Asthi	8	8	8
Sandhi	20	20	20
Dhamani	9	—	—
Total	**107**	**107**	**107**

2. According to the site
Sakthi - Legs- 22 .
Udara and *Ura*- Abdomen and Chest- 12
Bahu- Arm - 22
Prushtha- Back -14
Jatru-urdhva- Above clavicle- 37

3. According to size
1. One finger breadth (*Anguli Parimana*) - (Total 12).
2. Two fingerbreadth - (Total 6).
3. Three fingerbreadth -(Total 4).
4. Fist size or Four-finger breadth - (Total 29).
5. One Half finger breadth - Rest all (Total 56).

4. According to symptoms - when injured
Sadyha Pranahara - 19
Kalantara Pranahara - 33
Vishalyghna - 03
Vaikalyakara - 44
Rujakara - 08

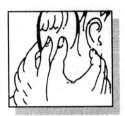

4.
Ayurvedic Physiology

Biological Humors -*Tridosha*

There are three main causative factors in the external universe: the sun, the moon, and movement (or wind). The sun, or the energy of conversion, is represented as fire; the moon, or agency of cooling and interlinking, is represented as the combination of earth and water; and wind, or the principle of propulsion, is due to the combination of air and ether. All the natural phenomena observed in the universe are caused by

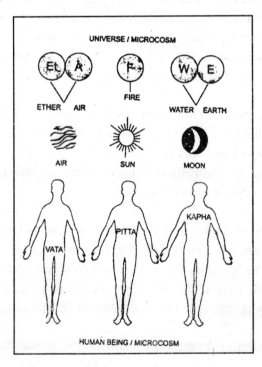

one of the three energies: 1) the agency of propulsion, 2) the agency of interchanging, or 3) the agency of cohesion.

The energy of propulsion causes the change in position of all things in the Universe-such as dust, smoke and clouds-in the direction in which the wind or force of propulsion is moving.

In human beings, the functions such as respiration, circulation, and elimination (the expulsion of waste products) are manifested as changes in position. Hence this energy of propulsion is called *Vata*. The Sun is bright red and yellow. When any substance comes in contact with the heat of the Sun, its temperature, form, appearance, or taste is changed. In the human body the same thermogenic energy changes the ingested food into tissues and waste products. This energy is known as *Pitta*. The effects of these two energies are inhibited by the third energy-the agency of cold and cohesion, which in nature produces rainfall. This force is responsible for new growth, hence it is named *Kapha*.

According to Ayurveda, these three primary life forces are called Biological Humors, or doshas, and the science of these three is known as tridosha. These humors, being very subtle substances, are the primary forces behind all physiological and psychological functions.

The biological air humor is called.Vata, and means "that which moves things." It is the motivating force behind the two other humors. The biological fire humor is called Pitta, which means "that which digests things." The biological water humor is called Kapha, which means "that which holds things together."

All the activities in the universe or in the human being are classified according to three basic functions: creation, organization, and destruction. These are the functions respectively of the three main Hindu Gods, *Brahma*, *Vishnu*, and *Shiva*. The *Tridosha* theory names these three functions after the three biological humors or *Doshas*. Pitta, the thermogenic humor, organizes body activities after conversion. Kapha, the cohesive humor, is responsible for maintaining the creation. Vata, the bio humor for air, controls destruction.

Properties of *tridosha*
Vata is recognized by its qualities of dry, light, mobile, agitated, cool, rough, less- nourishing, propulsive, and subtle. It possesses an astringent taste. When the living body comes into contact with substances of such qualities, it loses bodily constituents. Even though these qualities are harmful to existing tissues in the body, they are essential for body functions. If subtlety in the structure of a tissue is nullified, there will no movement in it at all.

Pitta is slightly oily, sharp with an unpleasant odor, light, and fluidic (liquid, flowing in some direction) with secretory and vasodilating properties. It has penetrating and hot qualities, and is pungent and sour in taste. In the process of digestion it is an easily flowing fluid. All colors except white and dusky or violet denote existence of Pitta.

Kapha is wet, oily, cool, smooth, sticky, dull, heavy, nourishing, slimy, compact (dense), white in color, and both sweet and salty by taste.

Functions of the doshas
Functions of Vata
Vata, as the principle of propulsion, carries out many diverse

functions in the human body. It controls cell division and arrangement of cells and their formation in different layers. It conducts afferent impulses from special sensory organs (*Jnanendriyas*) to the brain and efferent impulses from the brain to motor organs (*Karmendriyas*). Vata controls the expulsion of feces, urine, sweat, menstrual fluid, semen, and the fetus. It also controls the respiratory, cardiac, and gastro-intestinal movements, as well as all higher functions in the brain and spinal cord. Vata controls the mind and gives the energy to perform all bodily activities-subtle and gross-as well as mental activity.

Functions of Pitta

Pitta is responsible for the formation of tissues (*dhatu*), waste products (*malas*) and energy (*doshas*) from the food, water, and air that we take in from the outside. It controls metabolic (both anabolic and catabolic) activities. It is responsible for all the secretions in the gastro-intestinal tract, and the enzymes and hormones from the ductless glands entering the blood stream. It controls body temperature, as well. Sensations of hunger, thirst, fear, anxiety, anger, and lust are all controlled by Pitta. Pitta is also responsible for actions of bravery and the assimilation of all knowledge from the outside.

Functions of Kapha

Kapha increases the deposits in the cell mass as well as the destruction of tissues from wear and tear by maintaining the strength and immunity of the body. The capacity for reproduction, zest, and correct retention of knowledge depends upon the proper function of Kapha. It is essential for the interlinking of cells, tissues and organs. It is thus responsible for the growth of the body.

Types

Vata
1-2. *Prana-Udana*

These two are exactly opposite movements and are taken together. Although the function of *Prana* can be studied at the level of brain, heart and lungs, generally speaking its movement is from outside to within and forward. Pranic propulsion is responsible for receiving substances-like air, water, food, and knowledge-from the outside world through

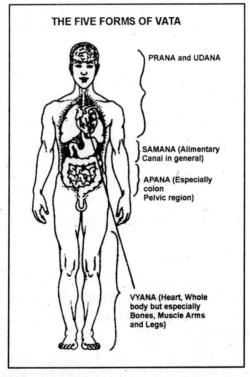

THE FIVE FORMS OF VATA

PRANA and UDANA

SAMANA (Alimentary Canal in general)

APANA (Especially colon Pelvic region)

VYANA (Heart, Whole body but especially Bones, Muscle Arms and Legs)

the five sense organs.
Udana propulsion is from inside to outside and upward,

23

mainly as expiration. Speech is due to *Udana*, and remembrance is the bringing out of knowledge that has been put in by the *Prana*.

3-4. Vyana-Samana

Vyana is responsible for propulsion from center to periphery. The movement of the heart and the propelling of nutritive substances to the periphery is the function of *vyana*. It is also responsible for the movement of limbs and the flow of the blood and sweat.

Samana, on the other hand, is the propulsive force from periphery to center. Bringing all the fluid back to the heart, impulses from the different organs to the brain, and propelling all fluids into the lumen are the functions of *samana*.

5. Apana

In contrast to the two pairs above, the function of *apana* is to control the movements of constituents like urine, feces, menstrual discharge, seminal discharge, and flatus. All these are controlled for a particular period of time before being discharged from the body. The overall control of all these substances for such a period is beneficial to building or maintaining the tissues. Since this control is beneficial to other types of Vata, it is said that apana controls the different forms of Vata.

Pitta

The five types of Pitta are *Pachaka, Ranjaka, Alochaka, Sadhaka,* and *Bhrajaka.* All of these are responsible for some type of conversion.

1. *Pachaka -* is responsible for the primary conversion of food in the Gastro-Intestinal -Tract. It is responsible for conversion

24

of external primordial elements in the food to the bodily primordial elements. Because of its hot and penetrating quality it disintegrates and digests food in gastro-intestinal tract.

2. *Ranjaka* - helps in the secondary digestion of food for the

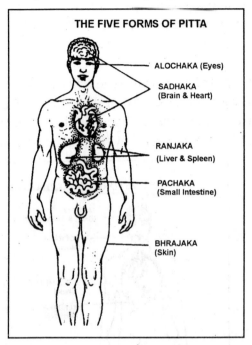

THE FIVE FORMS OF PITTA

ALOCHAKA (Eyes)

SADHAKA (Brain & Heart)

RANJAKA (Liver & Spleen)

PACHAKA (Small Intestine)

BHRAJAKA (Skin)

formation of tissues. The formation of blood (*rakta*) and other tissues in the liver is the chief function of *ranjaka* pitta.

3. *Alochaka* - is responsible for the digestion and conversion that takes place when an object is being sensed by the eye. (This is observed in the mechanism responsible for photosensation.)

It is inferred that the sensations of sound, touch, taste, and smell also involve a certain form of conversion for which the *alochaka* Pitta is the factor responsible for this conversion. .

4. *Sadhaka* - is located in the brain. After sensing an object, its real and quick understanding (comprehension) is dependent

upon a specific sequence of conversions by *sadhaka* Pitta. The capacity to grasp and of creative art is the function of *sadhaka* Pitta.

5. <u>*Bhrajaka*</u> - is responsible for the conversion of oils and ointments applied to the skin and maintain the temperature and complexion of the skin.

Kapha

The five types of *Kapha* are *Avalambaka, Kledaka, Bodhaka, Tarpaka,* and *Shleshaka.* All of these protect various organs from wear and tear due to Vata and the hot and penetrating effects of Pitta. Similarly they help in the cohesion and

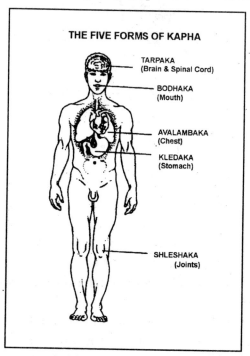

THE FIVE FORMS OF KAPHA

TARPAKA
(Brain & Spinal Cord)

BODHAKA
(Mouth)

AVALAMBAKA
(Chest)

KLEDAKA
(Stomach)

SHLESHAKA
(Joints)

interlinking of tissues.

1. <u>*Avalambaka*</u> - protects the lungs, heart, and proximal part

of the intestines. Due to repeated contraction and relaxation, the lungs and heart are subjected to substantial wear and tear. But the fine slimy and oily secretions inside these organs protect them and maintain their integrity.

2. *Kledaka* - protects the upper and middle abdomen from hot, irritant, or cold food as well as from the secretions of *pachaka* pitta.

3. *Bodhaka* - protects the mouth from pungent, hot, cold, or irritating food and drinks. It is responsible for experiencing the various tastes of food. *Bodhaka* guards mouth by initially rejecting potentially harmful substances.

4. *Shleshaka* - lubricates all the bony ends of the joints and protects them from friction, during movements.

5. *Tarpaka* - provides various nutrients to the brain cells and gives lubrication and protection to the brain and spinal cord.

Tissues and Waste Products

The dhatus, or tissues, are the constituents, which do not get eliminated from the body (except the reproductive), and they remain well within a particular limit. This limit is the skin from the outside and the internal linings-of the gastro-intestinal tract, bladder, joints, cerebral linings, etc.-from within the body. As the body strength increases these tissues go on developing. They are seven in number.

Function of tissues

1. Plasma provides nutrition to all tissues and gives sense of pleasure, happiness and contentment. It is responsible for hydration and maintaining electrolyte balance of the body. The term *rasa* means to circulate.

2. Blood is particulate matter e.g. R.B.C.; W.B.C.; etc. Apart from giving *Prana* or vital force (oxygenation) to all tissues,

it is also responsible for love and faith. The term *rakta* is to give color.

3. All the muscles in the body provide binding, covering to inner structures and gives strength to body frame. The term

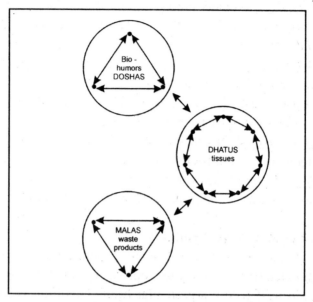

Dosh - Dhatu - Mala

mamsa is derived from the root '*mam*' meaning to hold firm.

4. The function of adipose tissue is lubrication (*snehana*). *Meda* means what is oily.

5. The function of asthi is to support the body. The term '*asthi*' is derived from the root '*stha*' to stand or to endure.

6. The function of nerve tissue is to give sense of fullness, contentment, and to fill empty spaces, in the bones and cavity inside the skull.

7. The function of reproductive tissue is not only to produce another life, but also provides strength, energy and stamina. '*Shukra*' itself means seed or luminous. It has two

components - a) seed element - semen and ovum and b) pleasurable fluids released during sexual activity. In men both these components function together, while in women the work separately.

Waste products (*mala*) are the constituents that are constantly being eliminated from the body. Their physical appearance varies from gaseous, liquid, semi-solid, to solid form.

The gross waste products (*sthoola mala*)- are urine, feces, and sweat. Although they are malas, they also have to carry out important function in the body before they are eliminated from the body.

Name	Function
1. *Purisha* -feces	a) Providing support to the agni.
	b) Giving support and strength next to tissues.
2. *Mutra* - urine	Collecting all the *kleda* from different channels and their elimination.
3. *Swedà* - sweat	Elimination of *kleda* from the skin and holding some part of kleda for giving moisture to the skin.

The subtle waste products (*sookshma mala*)
They are known as *Kleda*. They are produced in the respective channels of tissues. These are exudations eliminated from the epithelial linings of the eyes, nose, mouth, ears, and genital organs. Similarly, many minute waste products that are formed in the body during tissue formation from food are also considered in subtle waste materials. Health is maintained when these waste products are eliminated properly. When they accumulate in excess, various diseases are produced.

29

5.
Constitution-*Prakruti*

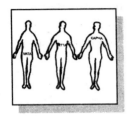

Definition

The predominance of elements, gunas, and doshas at the time of fertilization decides the constitution or bio-typology of that individual. Once this proportion is set it generally remains permanent for the life span of the individual. Class, family traits, locality, time, age, and individuality also influence the physical constitution.

The predominance of elements decides the physical constitution, while the predominance of *gunas* decides the psychological constitution. The predominance of humors (doshas) determines the Doshic *Prakruti*-the functional, or the energetic, condition of the body.

Doshic-Functional-Constitution
With the permutation and combination of the three doshas,

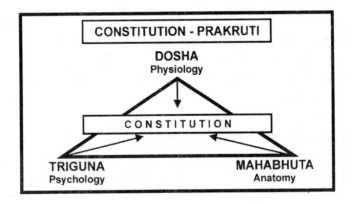

seven types of constitutions are formed:

a) Single dosha predominant- 1) Vata, 2) Pitta, 3) Kapha,

b) Duel dosha -4) Vata-Pitta, 5) Vata-Kapha, 6) Pitta-Kapha, and

c) Balanced constitution (*samaprakruti*).

These types are classified by their predominant factor. We find that a purely single Dosha constitution is seldom found and although a balanced constitution is extremely good, this type is also rare. (Many scholars have classified constitution in 10 types. They include the other three type - Pitta-Vata, Kapha -Vata and Kapha- Vata).

The Vata constitution is usually inferior in terms of health and longevity, Pitta is usually in between, and Kapha is usually superior. Of the duel constitutions, the Pitta-Kapha type is difficult. *Samaprakriti*, or the constitution, in which all three doshas are in equal proportion, is best.

Vata Constitution

Those of Vata constitution usually have tall or thin body frames and less strength. Their body weight is low and they have less resistance to disease. Their digestion and metabolism is changeable, hence they cannot form sturdy and stable tissues. Their life span is usually shorter than that of other individuals. Because of this variable nature in constitution, they cannot perform tasks steadily and continuously. Consequently they may fail in achieving their goals.

Such individuals require a job with little or no strenuous physical activity, in which constant attention is not required, and which is not in a cold or air-conditioned atmosphere. If they are forced to undertake such work they are likely to develop diseases of the nerves and bones, and to suffer from constipation along with loss of weight.

31

Pitta Constitution

Those of Pitta constitution have rapid digestive and metabolic activity. Thus they require constant food and drink which is cool and oily in nature. They are able to convert food into good quality tissue, but as the total conversion rate in the body is very fast, they also usually have shorter lifespan as compared to others.

They have soft, oily, and smooth skin. They tend to become bald at an early age, and their hair becomes gray prematurely. They have moderate strength and capacity to work, although they are hot-tempered. They are very intelligent and possess an excellent capacity for comprehension of concepts. They usually possess good knowledge any subject that interests them, and are creative in nature.

These persons require a job in a cool atmosphere, with some creative activity and intelligent work. They should not deal with chemicals, dyeing material, or petro-chemical substances, nor work near heat.

Kapha Constitution

Those of Kapha constitution possess hefty, robust, and thick body frames with good stout musculature. They naturally possess good strength, immunity, and vitality, and have a longer life span with good health. They have smooth and deep voices, and are often good-looking. The total digestive and metabolic rate in these individuals is very slow, hence they require less food and drink. They are of a calm and quiet nature.

Kapha types can carry out work that is heavy or strenuous. They are also good in maintaining public relations. However they should not work in cold and damp atmospheres. They are likely to become obese and become sick with joint diseases and heart problems.

Evaluate your Uniqueness - *Prakruti*

To asses your *Prakruti*, fill out the following form and mark the answer according to your own personal long term nature. If two answers apply for the same question, mark them both. If none is applicable leave it blank. Then tally each column. The column with the most marks is your *Prakruti*, the column with the second largest number is your secondary *Prakruti*. For example if you score 18 Vata, 7 Pitta and 4 Kapha: then your *Prakruti* is Vata-Pitta.

Vata	Pitta	Kapha
Physical characters		
Body frame lean, tall or short	medium	short, heavy
Musculature wiry, thin	smooth, flabby	robust
Skin dry, rough	soft, medium oily	thick, oily
Veins, tendons exposed, wiry	covered, soft	well hidden
Skin temperature cold hands, feet	warm	cool
Hair dry, rough, kinky	soft	thick, oily
Complexion dark brown, black	pinkish	pale, whitish

Teeth		
small, carries	medium	large, healthy
Gums		
thin, receding	easy to bleed	strong

Physiological Characters

Appetite		
variable	strong	low
Thirst		
less	always thirsty	less
Bowel movements		
constipated	normal	regular
Voice		
dry, high pitched	melodious	soft
Speech		
fast, talkative	authoritative	pleasant
Stools		
dry, hard	soft - loose	soft, thick
Urine		
less	normal	abundant
Menstruation		
painful, irregular	heavy, regular	normal
Sexual drive		
variable	passionate	strong
Strength		
fair	better	excellent
Exercise tolerance		
low	better	good

Psychological Characters		
Mental activity quick, restless	sharp, aggressive	calm, quiet
Thoughts too much, changing	steady, pointed	steady
Concentration good for short time	better	always good
Sleep light, interrupted	sound, medium	sound, heavy
Dreams flying, fearful	fiery, violent	water, calm
Grasping power quick	medium	slow
Memory short term -good	good	longterm good
Total **VATA**	**PITTA**	**KAPHA**

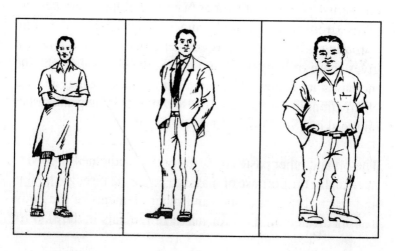

35

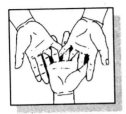

Action of Massage

For massage, the word used in many Ayurvedic texts is '*samvahana*' The word *mardana* has also been used as synonym to this. The term *mardana* means massage including pressing, rubbing and also includes other procedures like manipulation of muscles, hairs and joints.

It has been divided in various types like i) *deha samvahan-* or *deha mardana-* whole body massage, ii) *Kesa mardana-* head massage. iii) *Udvartana* -massage to the body with dry powders, iv) *utsadana* -massage with herbal paste v) *udgharshana-* reinforced massage with dry powders, and vi) *abhyanga* - massage with oils. (*Vatsyayana* 1-3-15)

Sushruta has mentioned that *udvartana* or massage with dry, hot herbal powders alleviates Vata and Kapha, reduces fat, gives strength to the body and is beneficial to the skin. *Utsadana* is more useful as cosmetic massage in women. It gives sense of happiness, and makes the skin soft, light and increases its beauty. *Udgharshana* is useful for removing obstructions in the channels. It also removes itching and rashes on the skin. (Su. Chi.24/ 51-43)

The oil and other pastes of herbs or the medicines applied to the skin for the purpose of massage permeate through the skin and reach different tissues and other elements of the body. The medicated oil used for massage remains in the skin for

300 (matras or) seconds and then gradually spreads to *rakta, mamsa, meda, asthi* and *majja*. The oil takes 100 seconds each to pervade thorough these tissues. (*Sushruta*)

Biological air humor or Vata dosha is located in *sparshnendriya* - sense organ of touch - and this is located in skin. *Abhyanga* is conducive to the healthy growth of the skin. The word '*abhyanga*' is literally derived from the Sanskrit root - *abhyanj* - (*abhi+anj*), that means to anoint or smear. Of all the sense organs the sense organ of touch is the most pervading and it has inseparable association with the mind. Hence the effect of massage is not only for controlling Vata dosha but it has its effect on the mind also. *Abhyanga* followed by *udvartana* and fomentation removes obstruction from the srotasas or the channels. *Abhyanga* and *mardana* also helps to prevent old age and the wrinkles on the skin.

Proper massage with oil removes dirt from the skin cleans millions of pores on the skin and helps indirectly to the action of lungs, large intestine and kidneys. With massage the blood circulation gets increased and this helps the exfoliation of superficial dead skin cells, tones the skin and encourages its rejuvenation process. Massage also helps the skin to maintain its elasticity and strength. Increase in blood circulation helps to acclerate the lymphatic system, which absorbs and eliminates many waste products.

Even if the idea of massage might be attractive, enjoyment of massage is not something that is immediately acceptable to everyone. There are many reasons for these, if you were not handled agreeably as a child, you are unlikely to trust being handled as an adult. Fortunately the body is designed in such a way as to be constantly massaging itself and this can give us some confidence to being with. The diaphragm muscles between the chest and abdomen alternatively compress and release the digestive organs with each deep breath. Even the slightest movement of the limb muscles squeeze and receive pressure on the nearby veins to keep peripheral circulation flowing. The arms, kept free to swing by the sides as we walk, relax the muscles at the back. If we are able to imagine this we are on the way to appreciating the advantages offered by applied massage. In order to gain full benefit, you need to be totally passive and surrender to the touch of skilled masseur or therapist.

There is great deal of evidence that the state of mind and nervous system is reflected in the state of musculature. Depending on the depth of the masage and various types of movements used by the masseur, the nerve endings can be stimulated or soothed. Similarly, massage or bodywork is one route into sunscious mind.

Human beings need to touch and be touched. Great deals of animal and human research shows that individuals deprived of physical contact are insecure, poorly adjusted and more prone to illness.

Massage is a very sensitive and sensitizing form of human contact, whose medium is touch, a sense to which animals as well as human being's are especially responsive. The first experience of massage is obtained when the fetus is delivered from the uterus due to rhythmic contractions of the uterine muscles. After we are born, holding, rocking, washing and caressing by the parent prepares our body for its independence.

Animals also are aware of the action of massage on their

newborn. Hence many animals lick the entire body of the newborn immediately after the birth. This helps not only to clean there body but gives them soothing massage with the tongue.

Massage increases the blood circulation and improves the nutrition. It has been shown by various scientific experiments, that more blood flows through the tissues during and after the friction or rubbing. Some experiments have also shown that the number of red blood cells also increase after massage. At the same time the flow of lymph also gets accelerated.

The waste products like lactic acid and congestion of blood in the exhausted muscles gets removed, hence they become refreshed. Massage also improves local and general nutrition of the body.

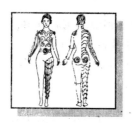

7.
Basic Strokes of
Massage

Massage Techniques

Massage is not just rubbing or pressuring if the body or application of oil alone. For full benefit from massage one needs to understand the systematic way of doing massage.

1.Friction -(*Gharshana*)

This is also called as 'connective tissue massage'. This can be done by thumb, fingertips, knuckles or palm of the hand. To improve the blood circulation of the body this is very useful. In friction massage, more pressure is applied on muscular part while gentle pressure is given on the bony parts. Thumbs

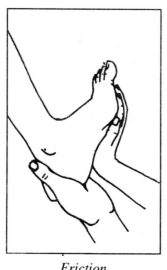

Friction

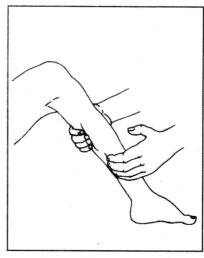

Friction

and palms of both hands are used for friction.

There are following sub- types of friction -
a) Towards the heart (*partiloma*) -This should be done on hands and legs by using pressure of thumb or palm of the hand. For treating varicose veins it is very useful.
b) Away from the heart (*anuloma*)- this type of massage is done for the whole body massage.
c) Circular - Mainly for the big muscles on hands and legs. Holding hand or leg in one hand and giving circular pressure by the other hand should do this. Carry out this technique from palm to shoulder or from sole of the feet to hip joint.

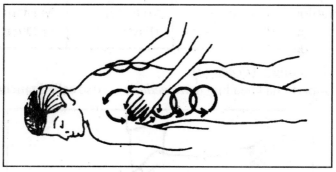

Circling

d) Zig-Zag - On the spinal cord or sternum from downwards to upwards it is useful by using fingers or palm of the hand.
e) Round - Useful in flat surface or joints for Vata-Pitta or Kapha type people.

Following rules are applied for friction

Direction	Pressure	Frequency Per minute	Material used
Vata anuloma	Moderate	30 to 60 (Slow)	Sesame
Pitta anuloma	Gentle	60 to 90 (Moderate)	Coconut or sunflower
Kapha pratiloma	Deep	90 to 120 (Fast)	Mustard or Olive

2. Kneading - (*Peedana*)

a) Superficial kneading (*avapeedana*) - Also called pinching.

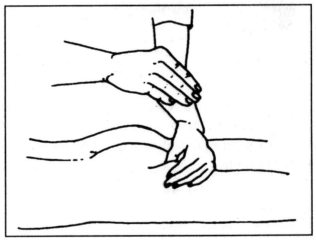

Pinching

By using thumb and index finger skin is lifted and pinching is given. Useful for improving the peripheral or capillary

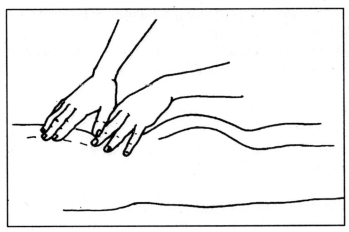

Feathering (Anguli Peedan)

circulation. Given in any direction. But it is different from lymphatic massage. This is useful in skin diseases.

b) Deep kneading (*pra-peedana*)- This type can be divided into several types as below-

Petrissage - By using palms and giving parallel deep pressure to the part of the body. This method is mainly useful for muscular part of hands & legs to improve deep and superficial circulation.

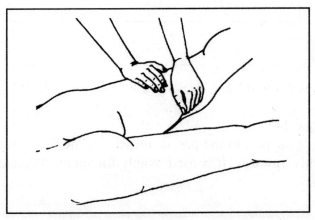

Rounding

i) Palmer kneading - By using palm over abdomen back and chest this type of kneading is done.

ii) Fist kneading - Used mainly on abdomen. This method is useful for relieving chronic constipation.

iii) Digital kneading (*anguli peedana*)- By using fingers and giving deep pressure, this type is useful for back, face etc.

3.Rounding

This is very fast movement by using both hands. The objective is to move muscles in round direction.

4.Wringing or twisting (*Udveshtana*)

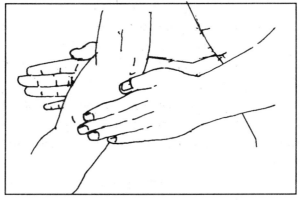

Rolling

The muscles are twisted by using both hands. In this type of massage, rolling and twisting actions are carried out.

5.Chucking

Giving support to the part of muscles while they are lifted slightly upwards. It is used mainly for sprain and catching pain.

44

6. Stroking - (*Trasana*)

Fingers and palms are used for this method by giving more or less pressure. This is useful for head, back, chest and abdomen.

a) Digital stroking - Very gentle massage to stimulate bony parts or bony prominence like forehead, tibia, and vertebral column. This should preferably done by using the tips of fingers.

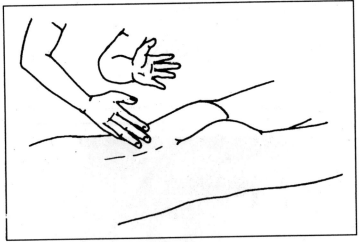

Stroking

b) Palmer stroking - Palms of both hands should be used on borders of the muscles of thigh, calf and buttocks.

c) Knuckle Stroking - By using back of fingers this stroke is given mainly where complicated muscles are there like chest and back.

d) Reflex stroking - to improve reflexes in diseases related to Vata and to improve activity of nerves, this is very helpful method.

7) Percussion - (*Praharana*) - Tapotement

In this type, the muscles or the body part is stroked by using the fingers or the palms of both hands. It is very useful for

Cupping

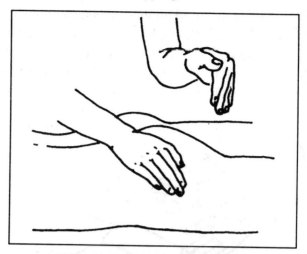

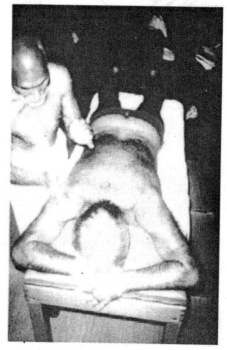

Tapotment

46

improving metabolism and local temperature of the body part. In Vata and Pitta type it is useful to remove obstruction to doshas and make the channel free.

Following types of Percussion are done -

a) Digital (*vadana*)- Using tips of fingers gentle strokes are given. Useful for head and chest massage.

b) Using palm of the hand (*aasphalana* or *tadana*)- useful for all over body.

c) By hand cupping (*samputaka*)- it is useful on muscular part of the body.

d) Pounding - done by using fists. Useful for heavy and strong

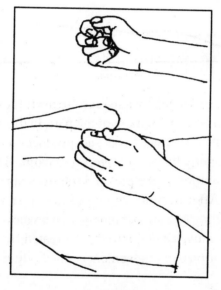

Pounding

muscles. It improves temperature and circulation of that part of the muscle or the body.

8) Vibrations (*Kampa* or *harshana*)

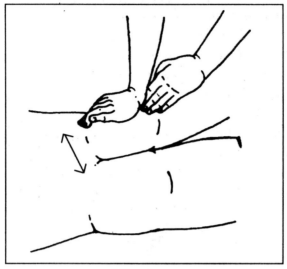

Vibrations

The vibrations produced by massage are useful for activating superficial and deep movement of the part. In this method the masseur vibrates his own hand and produces vibrations to the part of the body by using fingers and palm. This method improves circulation of the part and removes obstructions in the channels. After friction, vibrations are given to clean the channels. Tingling sensation, numbness, heaviness of the part, partial loss of muscles and atrophy is treated by superficial and deep vibrations and movement of the body part.

9) Joint movements - (*Sandhi Chalana*)

In this type the joints are moved and are massaged also. In daily life we observe that most people do not carry exercise hence movements of their certain joints are restricted and ultimately they become stiff. Massage with gradual increase

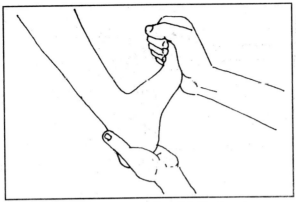

Joint movements (Sandhi Chalana)

in joint movements improves flexibility, removes congestion and helps free movements of joints. Please note that in case of frozen shoulder and tennis elbow this type of massage is associated with medicated fomentation.

Multiple movements are possible in hip and shoulder joints such as flexion, extension, abduction, adduction and circumlocution. Flexion, extension & rotatory movements are possible in ankle and wrist joints, while flexion and extension are possible in elbow and knee joints.

10) Touch - (*Sparsha*)

After completing all above types patient needs gentle touch for soothing effects. Hence it can be done all over the body or the part of the body to conclude the massage by giving very gentle touch by hands.

All these different strokes of massage were rationelized by Sweedish Professor Henry King in 19 th century.

11) *Mardana*

is usually done after *abhyanga*. In this method, gentle and suitable use of fingers, thumbs and palms are used for massage.

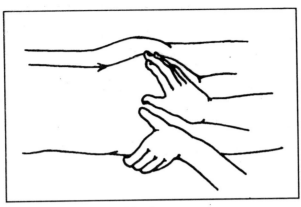

Mardana

Skill is more important than power. Patting, gentle rubbing, soft squeezing and vibrations are to be used. Movements are mainly to be performed according to the shape of the muscles. For Vata disorder and constitution - *Mardana* should be *anuloma* (in the direction of body hair and away from heart). For Pitta disorder and constitution - Combinations of *anuloma* and *pratiloma* should be used.

For Kapha disorder and constitution - It should be *pratiloma* . - towards the heart.

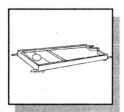

8

Ayurvedic Massage

In the chapter on history of massage, we have seen that practically every Country in the World has some kind of tradition of massage. In this context, often the question is asked that what is ite specialty of Ayurvedic massage ?

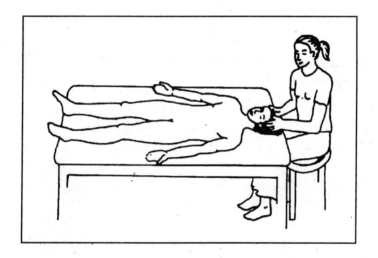

Ayurvedic massage has a long history as the part of Ayurvedic treatment. It is unique in the sense, that it is based on the principles of primordial elements, biological humors or *tridoshas*, and concepts of *agni* and Pitta, as well as the formation of toxins or *ama*. *Agni* is the energy, which represents the Sun in the Universe, and is responsible for all types of conversions in the body. It works through the medium of Pitta and is responsible for all the transformations - anabolic and catabolic. Thus for all digestive and metabolic functions agni is responsible.

When this agni becomes low, it is not possible to digest the food and other material properly which results in the formation of toxic substance called as *ama*. In the initial chapters we have learned some of these important principles.

The aim of Ayurvedic massage is to achieve the balance of energies inside the body and for this the study of the fundamental concept of *Prakruti* or your uniqueness is very much essential. To achieve this balance *Ayurvedic* massage uses varieties of substances like simple oils, powders of food substances like lentils, medicated oils, aromatic oils, and powders of various herbs. Also there are different types of massage, which vary according to the need of the patient and the disease he is suffering from.

In south India (kerala and Tamilnadu), some specific massage techniques have been developed as a result of tradition as well as research, which we have described in separate chapter. Various supplementary procedures like *Swedana (Fomentation), nasya, shirobasti, shirodhara* can be given along with Ayurvedic massage to enhance the effects. Ayurvedic massage also plays very important role in the treatment of rejuvenation or *rasayana* for achieving longevity.

Time of massage
Massage should preferably be done in the early hours of morning, when the stomach of the patient is empty. It can also be done in the evening, 3-4 hours after lunch. It should not be done immediately after taking food.

Ayurvedic types
Essential requirements

The room of the massage should be warm and cozy. Massage can be done either on the massage table, which is about the height of one's waist, or it can be also done on the floor. The table should be properly covered with clean white cloth, so that the patient is comfortable during the massage procedure. For other procedures like *taila dhara* - oil drip on the head- and massage special type of droni or table should be used which facilitates to recover the massage oil from the body of the patients. The masseur should be healthy, not suffering from any contagious skin disease and should cut all his nails properly, so that during massage they will not harm the patient. The oil to be used for massage should be cold during summer and warm during winter.

1. *Abhyanga*
means the application of plain or medicated oil to the body. The oil should be according to ones constitution, age, season, particular disease and atmosphere; to skin. For massage detail anatomical knowledge of *peshi, sandhi,* and *marma* is essential

Types of Abhyanga
1) Oil massage in Health,
2) Oil massage in different diseases,
3) Whole body massage,
4) Massage to some part of the body,
5) Self (Auto) massage.
6) Synchronized massage.

Abhyanga in health
Before *abhyanga* one should always ascertain his constitution as described in the chapter on constitution and then select proper oil for *abhyanga*.

Massage according to Constitution

Massage for Vata Constitution

Vata type people are dry, cool by nature - so oily massage should be given daily in the early morning or before a warm bath in the evening. The kind of oil massage lubricated dry skin and protects joints. Vata people are very sensitive to touch so warm oil is used. Sesame oil is best for alleviation - it removes dryness, coldness, stiffness and pain. Other medicated oils like dashamula oil-, which is, prepared from Ten roots- shaliparni (Desmodium gangeticum), prushniparni (Pseudarthria viscida), 2 types of bruhati (Solanum xanthocarpum and solanum indicum), gokshura (Tribulus terestris), bilwa (Aegle marmelos), shyonaka (Oroxylum indicum), patala (Sterospermum suaveolens), agnimanth (Premna integrifolia), kashamari (Gmelina arboria) and oil prepared from group of herbs included in *Jeevaniya* or *Brimhaniya* are the best for Vata. Similarly ashwagandha (Withania somnifera), bala (Sida cordifolia), narayana or mahanarayana (Asparagus racemosus) can alos be used. Vata massage oil is also usefull (see chapter 14)

Essential oils - ginger, basil, camphor, jatamansi and eucalyptus having hot potency are mainly used.

Massage for Pitta

These people have rapid metabolism and have tendency for fever and inflammatory disease. Their skin is sensitive and easily gets rashes or inflammed. So cooling massage oil should be used. Coconut and sandalwood oil is best for these people. Both these oils calm the mind and cool the body. Sunflower oil is also useful for inflamed skin. Medicated oils can be prepared from - ela (elettaria cardamomum), jatamansi, myristica fragrans, musta, chandana, nagakeshara and karpura.

Essential oils - lemongrass, lavender, jasmine, sandalwood etc. (See Pitta massage oil in Chapter 14)

Massage for Kapha constitution
These people have thick and oily skin. They need massage to improve their circulation and lymph drainage. Hence as far as possible oil should not be used. The best massage for these people is with the help of dry and hot potency powders of herbs with the use of very little oil, which is of hot potency like mustard or sesame. The massage should be vigorous and deep. It is preferable to use powders of calamus or vacha, dry ginger, dashamula and the powders of various lentils like chick pea or bengal gram. Medicated oils can be prepared with bilwa, dashamula, guggulu, shilajita, devadaru and tagara. Essential oils - Like basil, ginger, clove, eucalyptus can be used. (See Kapha massage oil in Chapter 14)

For persons of mixed dosha constitution
Vata-Pitta- should use less oil than pure Vata.
Pitta - Kapha - should use sunflower oil.
Vata-Kapha - should use dry powders of various hot herbs like acorus - vacha or dry powders of lentils and legumes like chic pea with small amount of hot and penetrating oils like mustard oil.

Self massage (Auto massage)
should be done by every individual, to maintain the health. Every person should use oil that is suitable to him according to his own constitution as explained above. There is saying in Kerala that person should use small amount of money on massage oils than giving large money to the doctors for curing diseases. This confirms that every day abhyanga, can prevent various diseases.

Massage oil,

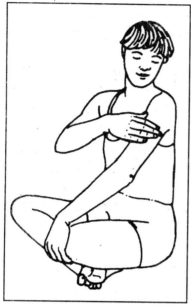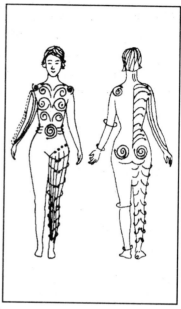

Self Massage

Hair oil,
Hot water bath,
Cleansing powder.

Procedure-

Usually different oils are used for head and for the rest of the body. Oils, which are cool in potency, should be used for applying on the head, while those, which are warming in nature, can be used for general massage. All most all oils since they are unctuous, heavy and warm act as Anti-Vata. Sesame oil is the best oil for Vata constitution and if properly processed, has anti-oxidant qualities.

Warm the required oil in water bath to 39 C. Sit on stool or chair in warm bathroom or other comfortable room. Pour the warm oil in your palm, so that you know the temperature of the oil.

1. First apply the oil on top of the head and massage the same for a minute. For massaging the scalp use the fingertips. Then massage the face, front and back of the neckand head with the palm. Give special attention to the head *marmas* like *adhipati, seemanta* and *shankha.*

2. Then take other oil suitable for the body massage, and start massaging the external ear by holding right ear lobe in the thumb and index finger. Use the tip of the index finger to massage the innermost part of the ear. Do the massage in the same manner to the left ear also.

3. Then start massaging the arms with back and forth movements and circular movements over the joints.

4. Now apply the oil to the chest and abdomen. Pour little oil in *nabhi marma.* On abdomen gentle circular movement should be used. Give gentle massage to the *marma* like *nabhi, basti* and *hridaya.*

5. Then apply the oil to the soles of the feet and then carry out the massage to the lower limbs. It is better to leave the oil on the body at least for 15 to 30 minutes. Then take warm bath or shower. Use cleansing powders of vacha- calamus or powders of lentils to take away the excess oil from the skin.

Benefits of *Abhyanga*

1. Beneficial to eyes- (*Drushti Prasad Kara*)- Proper massage around the eyes and face, makes eyes beautiful and shining. Increases activity of vision. Helps to keep away blindness and diseases of eyes. For treating disorders like myopia, massage to head (scalp) and feet (soles) is very useful. Massage to *kurcha* and *kurchashira marma* points is always beneficial for the eyes.

2. Nourishes the body - (*Pushtikara*) - Massage makes the

muscles strong. Increases stamina, vitality, and virility. It also helps for elimination of the waste products like sweat, urine, stool etc.

3. Promotes Longevity -(*Ayu Kara*) - The functions of vital organs and tissues can be improved and life span can be promoted through the practice of regular massage therapy.

4. Induces proper sleep- (*Swapna Kara*) - Physical and mental feeling of well being, nourishment, strength, sexual ability to perceive knowledge, depends upon proper sleep. Massage is a powerful agent, which induces sound sleep.

5. Makes skin soft and silky- (*Sutwak Kàra*) - Massage improves skin complexion and makes it shine and beautiful. It also resists premature wrinkles, unwanted hair and warts and increases immunity against skin diseases.

6. Makes the skin firm- (*Dardhya Kara*)- By properly removing waste products and providing nutrition, massage promotes sturdiness and strength of the skin.

7. Increases strength of the skin- (*Klesha Sahatwa*) - Massage increases the resisting power against physical and mental pressure, stress and strain, agonies, sorrows and anxiety. Improves general tolerance and patience.

8. Increases immunity of the skin- (*Abhighata Sahatwa*) - Massage induces speedy recovery of wounds and fractures and also resists permanent debility or deformity after fractures and accidents.

9. Removes fatigue- (*Shrama Hara*) - Overcomes fatigue. Fatigue due to routine work, mental stress, strain can be corrected by regular massage.

10. Regulates Vata- Prevents and corrects disorders by Vata or Nervous disorders. Vata regulates all the sensory and motor functions of nervous system and it also regulated the activities of Pitta & Kapha. Thus Vata plays most important role in the creation, sustenance, decay and destruction of the body.

Therefore for the individual to be healthy and happy, Vata must always be kept in equilibrium. Skin is the main sensory organ through which with the help of massage, Vata can be kept in equilibrium.

In short the secret of youth and beauty is the proper circulation of vital life fluids and the regular discharge of waste materials. For the above purpose massage plays very important role. Massage helps keep you feeling young, vital, beautiful and healthy.

The body is compared to tree. If the root of the tree is given water regularly then it lives for a long time. Similarly on the above analogy if a body of an individual is oleated properly through massage then he lives for a long time without any decay or disease.

Massage should be done regularly. As a person takes food daily so also he should resort to massage regularly every day. To a normal healthy person massage should be given before he takes bath. Massage is very helpful before performing physical exercise and is also useful for those who practice yoga. Massage should be performed only when the patient has digested the food taken during the earlier mealtime and when he is hungry and thirsty.

Mardana (light rubbing) should be followed by abhyanga. By gentle and suitable use of fingers, thumbs and palms massage is done. Skill is more important than power. Patting, gentle rubbing, soft squeezing and vibrations are to be used. Movements are mainly to be performed according to the shape of the muscles.

For Vata disorder and constitution - *mardana* should be anuloma type (in the direction of body hair and away from heart).

For Pitta disorder and constitution - combinations of *anuloma* and *pratiloma* should be used.

For Kapha disorder and constitution - It should be *pratiloma* type- towards the heart.

Therapeutic indications of *Abhyanga*

1) For general weakness- it is indicated from childhood to old age. It should preferably be given every day to remove wear and tear of the tissues, fatigue and to give strength to muscles and growth of body.

2) Disorders of joints - All types of arthritis i.e. osteo-arthritis (*asthigata Vata*), rheumatoid arthritis (*sandhigata Vata*), rheumatic arthritis (*amavata*), spondilytis, disorder of vertebral column and gout (*vatarakta*).

3) Diseases of muscles like myositis- means muscle inflammation with pain, spasm, atrophy, and various types of myopathies etc.

4) Nervous system disorder - Neuralgia - pain due to inflammation in the nerves, sciatica, poliomyelitis, hemiplegia, paraplegia and cerebral palsy.

5) Drug addiction - As a preventive and therapeutic in withdrawal syndrome.

6) Feminine problems - Dysmenorrhoea, oligo-menorrhoea, menorrhagia, leucorrhoea and menopausal syndrome. Massage after delivery to mother and child is done to relieve the Vata vitiation in mothers and to enhance the immunity in children.

7) Circulatory problems - After myocardial infarction, ischaemic heart disease, functional heart disease, cold hands and feet due to bad circulation, Varicose veins.

8) Disease in sportsmen - Tennis elbow, lumbago, frozen shoulder, shoulder and backache, sprains and aches etc.

9) Psychological problems - Schizophrenia, illusions,

depression, negative thinking, constant worry, loss of memory and insomnia.

10) Metabolic disorders - obesity, loss of weight and stamina, to increase digestive and tissue fire.

Contra -indications for *Abhyanga*

Person suffering from fever, indigestion and in those whom Panchakarma or cleansing treatment has been given.

Abhyanga in Therapy

Before therapeutic *abhyanga*, the physician or the masseur must examine the patient thoroughly to determine his constitution, type of disease, vitiated dosha, condition of ama (toxins) or nirama. Following form should be properly filled by them-

1. Examination of the patient

Name, age, sex, address.

History of chief complaints and their duration,

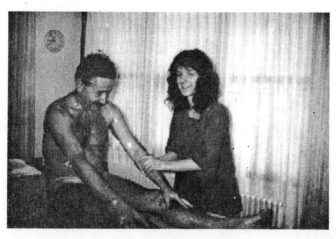

Abhyanga

Personal history about the allergy etc,
Family history,

General examination- this should include examination of tongue, urine, feces, pulse to determine whether the patient

has *ama* -toxins in his body or not. If the tongue is coated white, and this coating remains there even after scrapping the tongue, then it is clear sign that the ama is present. Similarly, if the urine is turbid with foul smell and the feces are foul smelling and they sink in the water; this also indicates that the *ama* is present in the body.

If the patient has toxins in his body, massage should not be given to him.

Later on systemic examination should be done to find out the type of disease and type of vitiated dosha. Oil for massage can be selected according to these findings.In this type one can carry out part or the whole body massage.

2.Requirements

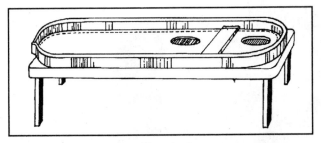

Droni

Massage Table
Vessel containing oils,
Hot water bath.

3.Main Procedure

Usually this is done in seven positions as follows-

1. First apply the cooling type of oil to the head and massage the head properly, while the patient is in the sitting position.

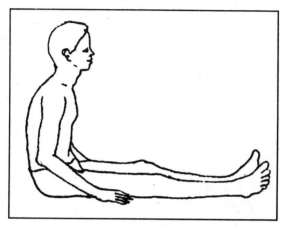

Give proper attention to *adhipati, seemanta* and other *marmas* in the region of head. Then take proper massage oil required for the body and apply the same to the ears, face, palms, and soles of the feet. Then start applying the oil on the neck and downwards on chest and back.

2. Ask the patient to lie on supine position on the back.

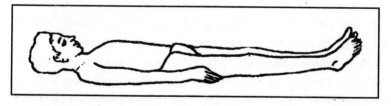

Foot Massage - the patient is lying on the table or on the

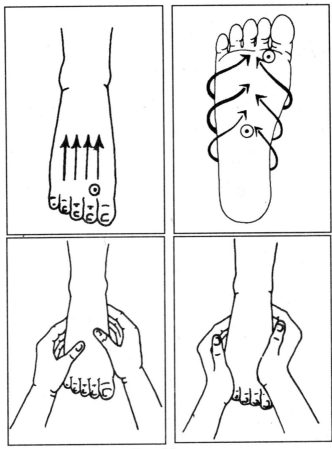

Foot Massage

floor. The masseur should stand or sit at the side of the patient. Apply plenty of oil to the sole of the foot, after cleaning the same with towel. Then make brisk *gharshana* - friction -on the sole of the foot and massage the dorsum of the foot. Stretch the fingers of the foot and massage them also.

Leg massage - Then apply oil from ankle to knee joint. Give friction massage to the calf muscles. Apply oil from knee to the groin, coming down with three or four rotary sweeps and with ocasional strokes with front and back of the fingers. Carry

64

out twisting, soothing and vibratory massage to the entire leg. The masseur should then raise the leg of the patient and keep it on its own shoulder and start rubbing from foot to hip with both hands six times at least. The masseur should then keep the leg down and flex the same at knee. Give circular massage to the ankle and knee joints.

Thigh massage- All the thigh muscles are big. They require kneading by fingers. Later on give pounding masage by fists also.

Massage to abdomen- The movement of massage on abdomen should be circular, and it should be light. Proper attention

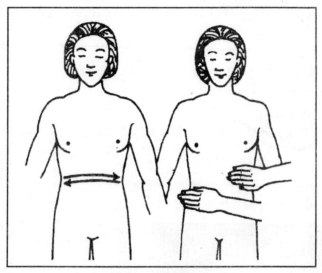

Abdomen Massage

should be given to the important marmas like hridaya, nabhi and basti.

Massage to the chest- Apply large amount of oil on the front portion of the chest. Start massaging at the level of last rib on each side and proceed upwards and inwards and then outwards and upwards. Then start from the midline of the chest and massage both the arms upto middle and back to the chest.

In case of females give circular massage to the breast. As far as possible do not touch the nipples during the massage.

3. Then ask the patient to take left lateral position.

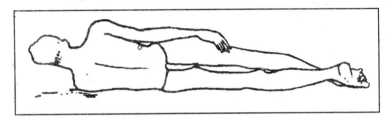

In this position, massage can be done to the right flank and right hand and feet also.

4. Ask the patient to lie on his back.

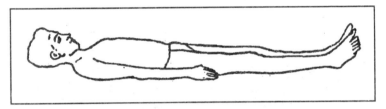

Hand massage - It should start from nails if the massage is

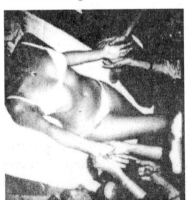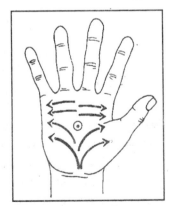

Hand Massage

being done for the cosmetic purpose. Put a drop of oil at the nail bed and give massage to the same. Apply oil to the palm and start massaging the front and back portion of the palm. Apply rotatory massage to the fingers and their joints. Then stretch the fingers slightly.

Arm massage- Apply the oil to the whole arm from wrist to the shoulder joint. Give circular massage on wrist, elbow and shoulder joints. Then give rolling type of massage to the entire arm by both using arms.

5. The patient should then take right lateral position.

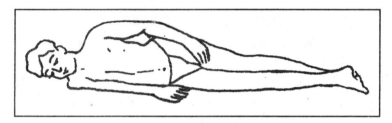

In this position, massage can be done to the region of left flank and left hand and feet.

6. Again ask the patient to lie on his back
and massage the chest, abdomen and both the extremities.

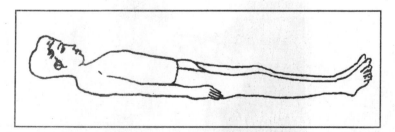

67

7. Lastly ask the patient to assume the sitting position

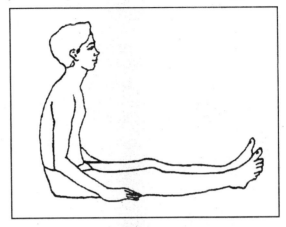

and massage all the body once again in this position.

Massage to the back - Unless and otherwise it has been specifically indicated, patient is not asked to lie on his abdomen, so that there is no excessive pressure on the abdominal organs. Hence massage to the back should be done in sitting and left and right lateral positions.

Neck Massage - Start massaging the vertebras from the

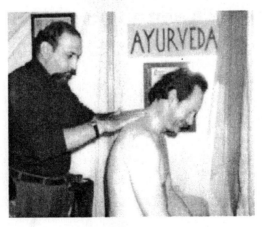

Neck Massage

cervical region and come down slowly to thoracic and then go to the lumbar region. Massage each vertebra with special attention to its ligaments and the muscles attatched to it.

4. Post procedure

After the massage patient can be given fomentation if it has been prescribed. Otherwise, wipe out the excess of oil with the help of applying dry powder or with the help of towel. Application of dry powders of vacha - calamus or other powders of lentils like chickpea is useful to wipe out excess oil from the skin. Then he is asked to take warm bath and then is allowed to take rest.

Synchronise masage

This is done by two masseures in simultenous and synchronised movements. The advantage of this type of massage is that both the sides of the patients are massaged at the same time. This gives maximum comfort and relaxation to the patient. The important part in this massage that both masseures must exert the same type of pressure while massage. They must have worked together for long time to achieve the effect of synchronised movements.

Massage to the Pregnant Women

For pregnant women massage should be given very carefully and it should be for as long as the women desires. If a regular massage is given to pregnant women it ensures painless delivery.

If the patient is lying down give her plenty of support with the help of cushions under her neck, back and at any other position she needs to feel comfort. For abdominal massage use light strokes. Apply sufficient oil all around the abdomen

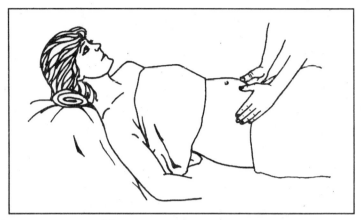

Massage to pregnant woman

and carry out soothing circular type of massage.

Female masseur should do breast massage. Due to this the *stanyavaha srotas* develops correctly and this helps in developing the nipple properly, so that the baby can suck the same properly and avoids cracking of the nipple.

For problems like backache, massage should be given to the back and at lumbar region in sitting position. Very gentle strokes and pressure is applied to entire vertebral column and back to relieve stiffness.

Massage to legs also should be done, which will relieve the problems of swelling of legs and varicose veins. Before labor and after delivery the women have some common complaints of, morning sickness, heartburn, sore breasts, constipation, sleep problems, stretch marks etc. in such cases choose a correct oil according to the constitution and give very gentle massage.

This should be complemented with a good diet and plenty of

rest.

Massage after delivery (Mother massage)

Immediately after the delivery, there is Vata vitiation in mother, as she looses lot of energy along with plasma and blood. There is much physical and mental strain on the body during the process of delivery. There is pain before and after the delivery due to the contraction of the muscles of uterus and other muscles in the area of back.

Massage helps the system to re-organize itself and also relieves the person. The child remains in the womb of the mother for the period of nine months, and due to this all the musculature on the abdominal region becomes stretched. After delivery, therefore there are white stretch marks on the skin of the abdomen called as stria gravidum. Regular massages after delivery not only helps to remove these but also give strength to the abdominal muscles, which can prevent hernia in this region. After 3 months of massage it helps the body to acquire the same shape as before.

This is done in the same style as of *abhyanga* and is preferably given in seven positions explained earlier.
Back massage is particularly done during labor.

Baby Massage

New born baby massage, is the old tradition of Ayurveda. After the cord is detached, the newborn and the mother receives massage every day with sesame oil or other medicated oil according to constitution.

Requirements-
Warm room,
Water bath,
Vessel containing oil,

71

Dry powder of calamus.

Benefits of baby massage
1. Stimulates circulation,
2. Gives good passive exercise,
3. Stimulates digestion,
4. Boosts immunity.
5. It was thought that the oil applied to the skin do not get absorbed in the
body. But now it is known that not only it gets absorbed but it stimulates various internal physiological functions also. Skin is the biggest organ of our body and proper massage by oils or medicated powders keeps Vata dosha in control.
6. It maintains and regulates body temperature, it also improves resistance
power.

Procedure

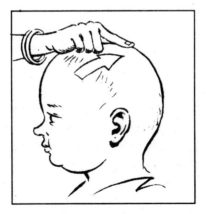

Baby Massage

Women masseur who knows this traditional massage usually

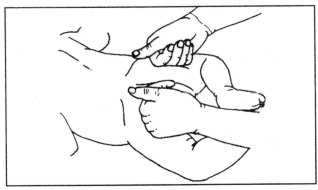

Baby Massage

gives the baby massage.

Position of the masseur- the women masseur usually sits on the ground with her legs stretched in front but are joined together. She then takes the baby on her lap and first starts purring warm oil on the anterior fontanel. A newborn baby instinctively responds to touch and massage. In newborn this place is very delicate, as the bones of the scull have not fused. Hence very gentle massage should be done with ample of oil putting in the hollow space here.

Later on put the baby in supine position on her back and give light strokes down to the chest and abdomen, gently stroking both hands and legs. While giving massage to the foot, slightly stretch the fingers and rub the foot. Later on massage the sole of the feet. Stretch the fingers of the foot slightly and massage them also.

Then keep the baby on her abdomen with face down and massage legs, back and hands as well. After 30 days medium pressure massage can be applied to the child. Squeeze both hands and legs and give passive exercise to both the extremities. For the back give gentle pounds and pressure by open palm. Finish the massage by soothing

73

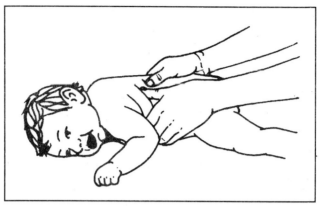

Baby Massage

<u>Post procedure</u>
After the massage, give warm bath to the baby. For removing excess oil, apply powder of Bengal gram or any other dry powder of lentils available. After bath quickly dry the body and apply powder of calamus on the head. The calamus is hot in potency and dry in quality, which prevents vitiation of Kapha and prevents cold and cough. Then wrap the body of the baby tightly in cotton cloth and allow her to sleep peacefully.

<u>For baby massage best-medicated oils are</u>
1.Bala oil- Bala in Sanskrit means child. This herb -sida cordifolia- is extremely useful in all disorders of children. The oil is prepared by taking bala juice, bala paste (*kalka*), sesame oil and cow's milk. (Baby oil by *Sewa*).
2. Chandan-bala-lakshadi oil, 3. Narayan oil, and 4. Baby massage oil (see chapter 14)

Udvartana
Means massage with pressure.
Two types - 1) Dry - With herbal powder massage (recommended in obesity),
2) Unction - Application of herbal paste (useful in debility).

Benefits-

It removes foul smell from the body.

It cures heaviness, drowsiness, itching, diseases caused by accumulation of waste products, excessive sweating and disfiguration of the skin.

It alleviates Vata.

It helps in mobilization of excess Kapha and fat.

It produces stability of limbs.

It promotes skin texture.

It improves the circulation in the channels.

It stimulates various doshas responsible for metabolic process in the skin, and keeps the skin healthy.

It specially promotes the complexion of the skin and also helps in removing unwanted hair from face and body.

Udgharshana

In this method, dry powders of medicinal plants are used and the massage is done by applying reinforced friction.

This type of massage has following benefits -

It cures itching, urticaria, and diseases caused by Vata.

It produces stability and lightness in the body.

It promotes the activities of *bhrajaka Pitta* in the skin and helps in removing sweat from the openings of the sweat glands.

Both these types of massage should preferably be done after abhyanga and mardana, before taking a bath.

For Vata disorders and constitution - Dry and coarse powders of amalaki (emblica officinalis), vacha (acorus calamus) and triphala are advised.

For Pitta disorders and constitution - Powders of sandalwood, musta (Cyperus rotundus), usheera (vetivera) and anantamula (Hemidesmus indicus) are beneficial.

For Kapha disorders and constitution - Use powders of haritaki, vacha, nimba (Azadirachata indica), and arjun (Terminalia Arjuna).

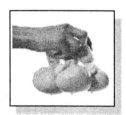

9.
Kerala Types of
Massage

1. *Chavitti*

Means feet. Compared to the massage by hands, feet can put lot of pressure on the patient's body. Hence this type is used for giving deep massage. This type is therefore more useful for robust Kapha type constitution people as well as for dancers and athletes for fitness and flexibility.

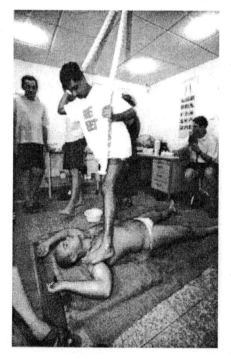

Chavitti

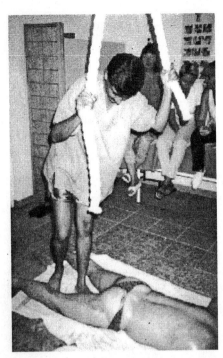

Chavitti

i) Preliminary procedure-

First the patient is given whole body *abhyanga*-massage- with suitable oil according to his constitution. Then he is asked to lie on the floor on warm carpet. A transverse rope is hanged for the support at the height of about 6 -7 feet depending on the height of the masseur. The masseur then takes hold of this strong rope while carrying out the feet massage. Instead of rope, masseur can also take hold of the rings attached to the ceiling and carry out the massage. At the side of the patient who is lying on the floor, a flat pan is kept. A suitable warm oil for massage is poured in this flat vessel.

ii) Main procedure-

Masseur then dips his foot in the oil and then starts massaging the patient. Like other types, this massage is also given for 30

77

to 45 minutes. *Charaka* has explained this procedure as *padaghata.*

iii) Post procedure -

After the massage, the patient is asked to take warm bath and rest at least for 30 minutes. He should avoid exposure to cold wind and should refrain from taking cold foods and drinks for the day.

2. *Pizhichil*

This is a combination of oleation and sudation therapy. *Pizhi* means squeezing and chil means vigorous synchronized movements (of massage).

i) <u>Requirements-</u>

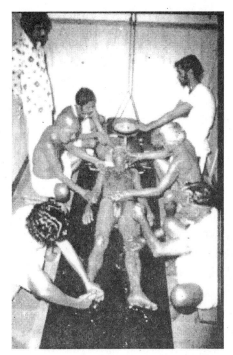

Pizhichil

78

In this type warm oil is taken in a pan. 8 to 10 fine cloth pieces of cloth are taken. These pieces are then soaked in the warm oil and squeezed over the affected part of the body.

ii) Preliminary procedure-

The patient is asked to lie on wooden *droni*. This is a special table prepared for this purpose. The table has the facility to collect the used oil for the purpose of massage quickly, which can be reheated and used again for the same purpose.

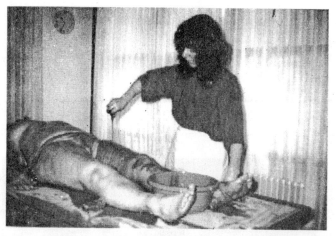

Pizhichil

iii) Main procedure -

As usual first gentle massage is given. Then this procedure is carried out 4 masseurs and they massage the patient with synchronize movements. At one time nearly 1 to 2 liters of oil is used for massage.

iv) Post procedure -

After 30 to 45 minutes, the oil on the body of the patient is taken out by applying flour of lentils and then he is asked to take warm bath. This type of massage is excellent for alleviating Vata dosha and hence used in the treatment of Vata

79

disorders. It also tones up the body and reduces fatigue.

3. *Uzhichil*
This is type of *abhyanga* in which special oils prepared according to Kerala tradition are used for massage. The requirements and other procedures are the same as that of *Pizhichil*.

4. *Navarakizhi*
or *shashti shalika pinda sweda-*
Requirements-
Massage table or wooden droni,
Cows milk 1 liter,
Decoction of bala (Sida cordifolia) 1 liter,
Navara rice 180 gms.
Procedure-

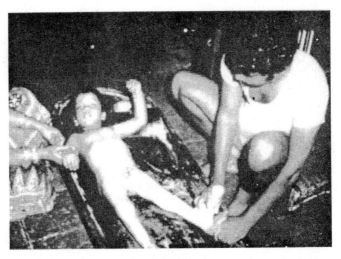

Navarakizhi

i) Pre procedure-
Navara is the special type of rice, which gets matured in 60

80

days. Cook the rice in the decoction of bala decoction. Cooked rice is then divided in 6 different equal parts and each one is put in piece of cloth. Then the edges are gathered and tied into a form of ball, which is then tied with thread. The bolus is prepared in such a way that the mouth of the sac has a tuft for holding it with ease.

ii) Main Procedure -

All the boluses are then kept in vessel containing *bala* decoction and this vessel is then heated.

The patient is then given *abhyanga* with suitable medicated oil and is asked to lie on massage table. Two masseurs then should start massaging the patient by holding the tuft of the bolus. As soon as the heat of the bolus is diminished, it should be replaced by the one which is warm and dipped in the decoction. This relay of warm boluses with cold ones should be continuously done till the decoction is finished. This massage with the warm bolus should be done in all seven positions.

iii) Post procedure -

after the massage, the paste of rice is removed from the boluses and that also should be massaged on the body of the patient. Later on it is gently wiped out from the body. Once again the oil should be applied to the patient and he should be allowed to take rest and then warm bath or shower.

Precaution-

The masseur on his own hand should taste heat of the bolus before applying the same for the purpose of massage. The relay of warm and cold bolus must be done in synchronized manner. As soon as the person gets good amount of perspiration, the treatment can be stopped.

This treatment can be carried out on alternate days for 7 to 14 days.

Indication-
Diseases of Vata, nervous system disorders, rheumatism, arthritis, muscular dystrophy, muscular weakness, paresis, paralysis and for general health.

Contra indications-
Excessive Kapha diseases, obesity, asthma and high fever.

5. *Kizhi*
Means poultice. Different poultices with various herbs are prepared according to the specific disorders like nervous and muscular or orthopedic complaints. Then with these poultices, massage is done. This is also known as *Elakizhi*.

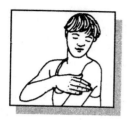

10.
Special care of organs by massage

Massage for Beauty

1) Face massage, 2) Head and hair massage, 3) Eye massage, 4) Ear massage, 5) Nose care 6) Foot massage, 7) Nail massage - nail care, 8) Vertebral column

1. FACE

There are 8 steps in Ayurvedic facial massage -
1) Cleansing, 2) massage with oils, 3) Herbal steam or compress, 4) gentle scrub, 5) Cleansing or Nutrifying mask/ facial pack, 6) toning/rejuvenating, 7) moisturizing, 8) hydrating, 9) Application of makeup (optional).

Cleansing, toning and moisturizing should be done every day. It is advisable to carry out full program once a week or at least twice a month.

Following are the benefits of facial massage

Enhances nourishment and cleansing of facial tissues, which gives glowing complexion to the face.

Maintains good tone and elasticity to all skin layers, which helps to hold youthful contours.

Melts away facial tensions and bodily stress, helps to remove wrinkles and brings gentleness to the expressions.

Redirects subtle energies.

1. Initial cleansing - Sweat and accompanying waste products constantly come out on the surface of the skin attracting dirt

and offering home to bacteria. Initial cleansing removes this dirt, making the skin surface fresh and ready to receive a facial massage. *Ayurveda* suggests the use of herbal powders called ubtans to cleanse the skin. The powders are mixed with liquids and applied as a thin scrub. All of these herbal powders improve circulation, sooth the skin and brings a glow to the complexion. For this purpose, powder of coriander, manjishtha, nutmeg, tulsi, sandalwood is generally used. They can be mixed with spring water, milk or aloe juice. These powders can be mixed with aromatic oils of rose and sandalwood, and then applied on the face, which is called an oil-based cleanser.

2. Herbal steams - The warmth, moisture and fragrance of herbal steam melts away muscular tension. It also helps to calm the mind and helps to remove stress and strain. Using steam is one of the oldest traditions in Ayurveda. The moisture softens the dry skin. The heat boosts facial circulation and activates the pores and glands, which brings the dirt and body toxins to the surface. To balance Vata dosha, oil can be applied after the steam. Frequency of steaming is determined by condition of the skin.

For dry skin - steam should be given once in two weeks. It is advisable to mix dashamula, rose or sandalwood powder with water.

For normal and oily skin - steaming should be done once a week.

For normal skin, it is preferable to mix ashwagandha and sandalwood, while for oily skin - lemongrass and rose powder is beneficial.

3. Gentle scrubs - A scrub should be very mild. It stimulates circulation. It brings a glowing luster to the complexion and

stimulates new skin growth. This can be done by using cotton or smooth cloth.

4. Nutrifying Mask - This extracts dirt from deeper layers of the skin preventing blackheads and acne. Muscles under the skin are nourished as they receive vitamins and minerals. This type of massage rejuvenates the skin, and has healing and soothing action on the skin. Masks can also stimulate the deepest layer of the skin to make new growth. Clay is the best base for a mask (gopichandan or multani mitti is used). It is a rich source of minerals. Aloe vera juice, lemon juice, or spring water is mixed with clay to prepare a mask.

5. Face packs - Face packs are softer and more porous types of facemasks. They improve circulation as well as clean and tighten the facial skin. Fruits and vegetables like orange, cucumber and fresh fruit juices are used to make face packs. Both masks and face packs should be removed with cool water and clean wash cloth.

6. Toners - It is useful to remove residue of all previous procedures. It tones ·
the skin. Using rose water, tulsi (basil) water as toner, this can be done.

7. Moisturizers - All types of skins need moisturizer. It protects the skin from heat and dry wind by acting as a physical barrier. It also protects skin from invasion by bacteria. Aloe vera, with glycerin, butter, ghee etc. is used as moisturizers. It is should preferably be applied at night.

8. Mists - A gentle touch of a spray mist brings vitality back to the complexion any time of a day. Mists are wonderful in

dry climate. Apply mist before and after moisturizing to assist absorption, it is made up of pure spring water. A heavy ring of metals like gold, silver is boiled in water & this water is used as mist after cooling.

Different techniques of facial massage -
Step one - Apply warm oil on both palms and start massaging with smooth strokes starting from midline of chin.

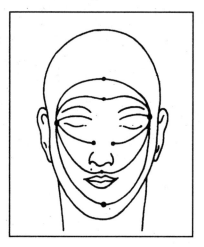

Step two - Place the fingers under the jaw, keeping thumb on jaw line. Ask the patient to open his mouth slightly and then manipulate the chin and jaw area by pressing up and releasing gently.

Step three - Place thumbs' on the jaw at the chin with index and third finger underneath the jaw line. Apply pressure to top and inner part of jawbone. Make light and small strokes in clockwise circles at temples.

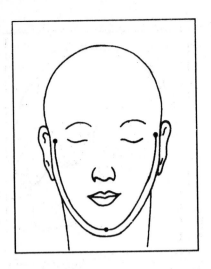

Step four - Place index finger between lower lip and tip of the chin. Ask the patient to open his mouth and make small clockwise circles at these points. Continue the massage from cheeks to temples.

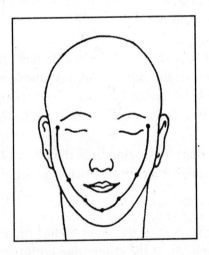

Step five - Place the tip of the index finger between nose and upper lip. This is the area of *shrungataka marma*. Press gently.

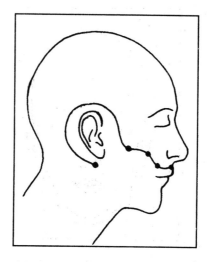

Then stroke from this point out on both sides up to the corners of mouth. Then under the chick bones to the top of the ear, over the ear, at the base of the ear where it touches the head to the bony bump (mastoid) behind the earlobe. Pay attentation to *vidhura marma* here.

Step six - Hold the left side of the patient's head with left hand. Place the right index finger just above the base of the nostril. Give small circular massage from this point up to the bony prominence behind the ear lobe but from over the ear.

Step seven - Start massaging from the midway between eyes and tip of nostrils. Direction of massage should be the same as above.

Step eight - Starting at the inner end of the eyebrow pinch along the eyebrow to the outer edge with the help of index finger and thumb.

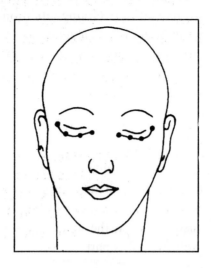

Step nine - Stroke from the tip of the nose to the area of third eye, which is between the eyebrows. This is *Sthapani marma*. Massage this area with gentle circle wise motion.

Step ten - Massage the forehead. Make zigzag motions from one side of the forehead to the other. Repeat this from right to

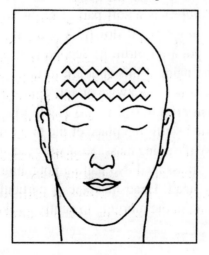

left and left to right. All types of techniques like pinching, pressure is given to all face. Giving vibrations to all face area later on soothing effect is given gentle touch.

Very gentle friction is very important in the case of giving massage to eyebrows, ears and nose. For friction some times smooth cloth or cotton is used.

2. HEAD

1. *Shiro Abhyanga* or Head massage -

The head is the center of the whole nervous system. It is the first organ, which is formed in the process of development of the fetus. The top of the cranium is called Brahmarandhra in yoga and is also known as the 'tenth gate'. Head massage is done very carefully to this part.

As we know all the important structures like cerebrum, cerebellum, mid brain, pons and the sense organs like eyes, nose, ears, tongue and skin are located in head. So massage of the head provides nourishment to all these vital organs and promotes their natural and normal functions. Also there are three important spots on the head.

i) *Brahmarandhra* is a soft part at birth- anterior fontanel, which later on gets hard slowly. A pad with oil or cotton is put on this spot after birth. ii) Second spot is where there is cowlick. The hairs at this spot are turning in the form of a whirl. Some times clockwise or anti clockwise. This area is also known as crest or *shikha*. iii) The third spot is where the neck meets the skull- the place of the brain stem or medulla oblongata. While doing massage on the head, these three spots are carefully massaged. No patting pounding or kneading is done on the head. Head massage is particularly beneficial before bathing in the morning to gently awaken the nerves.

<u>Head massage is especially useful for following</u>
It prevents and cures headaches.
It prevents and cures hair fall by making hair roots very strong.
It prevents and cures premature graying of hair.
It prevents and cures baldness.
It makes the hair long, soft and glossy.
It prevents and cures refraction errors of the eyes.
It endows a person with sound sleep.
Auto head massage done in the evening, helps remove the stress of the day and promotes peaceful sleep.

<u>Technique</u>
Start pouring oil on the top of the head. This oil is then spread all over the head by using fingers to the sides of the skull up

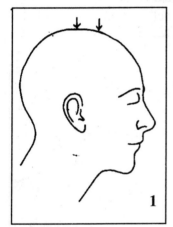 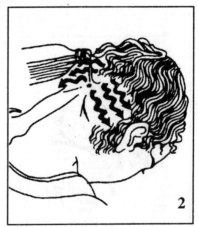

to the temples. Try to go along the *seemanta marma* points and massage the scalp. Then it should be poured on the second spot- shikha. By rubbing this oil all over the head hairs are twisted at the clockwise. Lastly press the head by two hands from forward to back and backward to forward.

When oil is applied to the head it gets absorbed in the scalp

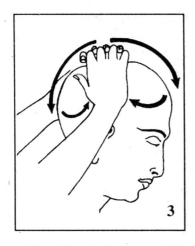 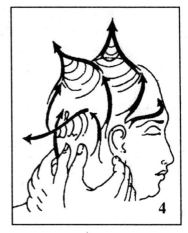

and reaches to the roots of the hair. This nourishes, lubricates and strengthens the hair roots and skin of the scalp preventing hair loss and premature graying. It helps to improve circulation

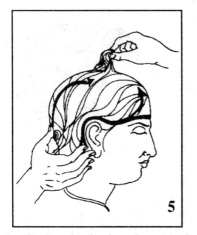 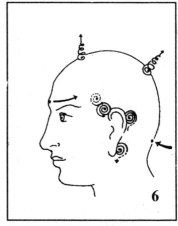

to the head relaxing the muscles & nerve fibers. This helps to refresh both the mind and the body. Relieving tension and fatigue. Massage to the head improves circulation of spinal fluid around the brain & spinal cord. It also increases the release of hormones and enzymes necessary for the growth of brain and relaxation of the body. Massage to the head

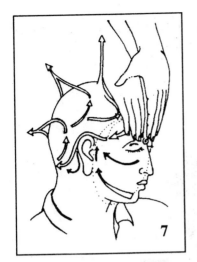 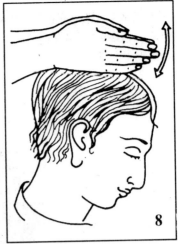

increases Prana, the subtle aspect of Vata dosha to the body. Massage to eyebrows and forehead improves eyesight and power of concentration. Head massage should be included in the daily schedule.

2. Shiro Dhara -

This is a process of running a fine stream of warm oil on the head, or forehead. It is one of the excellent therapies for the diseases connected with the head, neck, eyes, ears, nose, throat and nervous system. It's therapeutic utility is proven for Vata alleviation and for patients suffering from Vata diseases like insomnia and various mental disturbances. It is also used along with other medicines for the patients suffering from epileptic fits. During this therapy, medicated oil, milk or buttermilk is poured on the forehead between eyebrows.

If oil is used this therapy is called *tail dhara*
·If milk is used, this therapy· is called *dugdha dhara*.
If buttermilk is used this therapy is called *takra dhara*.

Technique -

Taila dhara - The patient is made to lie on his back on a wooden table prepared specially for this therapy. First *abhyanga* is done to the head. The patient's head is made to rest over a

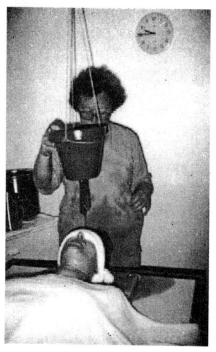

Shirodhara

slightly elevated position. Physician selects the oil (*taila*)to be used. For keeping oil, a special vessel is prepared having small bore at the bottom. Vessel is hanged and arranged above the patient's head. Oil is poured in the vessel and arranged so that the drip of the oil is constantly poured on the head. This therapy is given for 7 to 14 days and should be given early in the morning.

3. *Dugdha Dhara* -
In this method, stream of milk is poured on the head.

94

Medicated milk is used and is prepared by cooking the same with bala (sida cordifolia) and shatavari (asperagus racemosus). This is very useful for persons suffering from insanity, sleeplessness, giddiness and burning sensation.

4. *Takra Dhara* -

For this procedure a mixture of buttermilk with decoction of amalaki is used. This therapy is useful to cure premature graying of hairs, fatigue, headache, giddiness, burning sensation to palms and sole of the feet as well as for different types of disease of ear, nose eyes.

In short all types of dhara are beneficial as follows -

Alleviation of doshas in the region of head, neck, eyes, ear and nose.

Improving the functions of brain and central nervous system.

Maintaining calm and quietness of the mind.

Reducing stress and strain.

5. *Shiro Basti* -

Means keeping oil over the head with the help of tubular leather cap is called This is one of the important external oleation method.

It is indicated in facial palsy, insomnia, dry nose, dryness of eye, mouth migraine, headache, loss of memory, mental stress and strain and in Vata vitiation as well as Vata diseases.

i) Preliminary procedure- Shave the scalp properly. Give gentle massage to scalp and forehead and then give little fomentation to scalp, head and neck.

ii) Main Procedure - keep the leather cap over the head up to the ear lobes. Fill the gap within the head and cap by filling with wheat dough. Plastic mud can also been used for this purpose. Put warm sesame oil gradually.in the cap. It should be filled at least 4 inches above the scalp. This should be retained for 50, 40 and 30 minutes in Vata, Pitta and Kapha vitiation respectively.

Optimum signs of the procedure are secretions from nose and mouth and alleviation of the symptoms for which the procedure is undertaken. Once these signs are noted, oil is removed from cap.

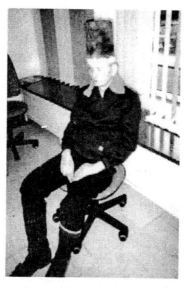

Shiro basti

iii) Post procedure -Afterwards ask the patient to take warm water bath. Advice the patient to avoid exposure to excessive cold, heat or dampness. Cover the head while moving out. Usually this procedure is done for 7 consecutive days.

3. EYE

Netra tarpana- (Netra basti)-

Means bathing eye with medicated oil. It is an ancient treatment from Ayurveda to release tension and to treat various eye diseases. This treatment is used to improve visual power as well as for the treatment of various other diseases like ptosis

96

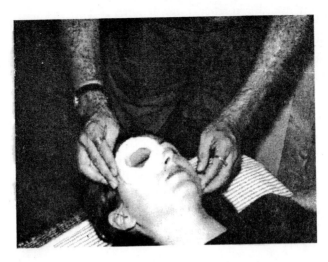

Netra basti

of eyelid, paresis of the muscles of the eye, squint due to muscular palsy etc. We have found that it also brings luster to the eyes, dryness of conjunctive, blinking of eye lids, enhances color and visual perception, creates sense of ease in the region of the eye. Due to constant work with computers, excessive exposure to bright light and television, there is stress and strain on the eyes and eyes gets fatigued and tired out very easily. For such problems Netra tarpana is extremely beneficial treatment. This treatment should be done in a calm, quiet and protected environment.

Requirement
Table
Vessel containing water
Vessel containing black gram flour or wheat flour

Technique
i) Preliminary procedure- First give gentle massage to the face, eyebrows and eyes by using very little oil.
ii) Main procedure - Form a round ring of two inches height,

around the right eye socket by using black gram or wheat dough. Pour warm cows ghee or medicated cow ghee in it. Ask the patient to carry out regularly open close lid movements of the eye. Depending on the vitiation of Vata, Pitta and Kapha; keep the ghee between 60 to 20 minutes. Afterwards remove the ghee by making a small indentation on the lateral edge (outer canthus) of the dough ring. If required carry out the process for the left eye also.

iii) Post procedure-After the treatment, wipe out the eye and then ask the patient to keep himself away from bright light and loud noise.

This procedure can be repeated for 7 days.

4. EARS

Massage to ears- like foot of the sole, the whole body is also represented on the pina of the ear. External massage to the pina of the ear is useful for treating various ear diseases.

Karna Purana

Means filling the ears with oil. By pouring the oil in to the ears, we can improve the function of the ear. Similarly several diseases, specific to this sense organ like wax in the ear, earache, deafness, tinitus, and several diseases of nearby organs like headache, lock-jaw, giddiness can be treated. This also corrects the diseases of gums and teeth. Ears and eyes are very closely related to the soles of the feet. Pouring oil in to the ears produces coldness and removes burning sensation in the feet. Pouring of oil in the ear should be done before meals during the daytime.

Technique

Hold the earlobe between thumb and index finger. Then with give rolling and gentle squeezing massage to outer edge of the ear. Also apply oil to the lobe. Then pour, warm sesame oil in the ear and rub the ear. Repeat the procedure in other ear.

Benefits
Facilitates improvement in circulation of the ear.
Helps to balance Vata dosha by having indirect effect on colon.
Stimulates brain.
Lowers blood pressure.
Absence of stiffness in chin and neck.
Absence of all ear diseases.
Removes dust and germs from internal ear.
In infection this massage should not be done.

5. NOSE -

Nasya
Means nasal administration of medicated powders or liquids. It is a procedure in which medication is administered through the nostril in order to purify the head and neck region. Here we use liquid drops that are more cleansing in action. By cleansing the sinus cavities, also head and neck region.
"Nasa hi shiraso dwaram" means nose is a door way to the head. Vitiated doshas above the region of claricle in the head-neck-are eliminated through nose. Hence this therapy is specifically advised for head and neck. Vata energy in the head is known as *Prana*. It is energy relates to higher cerebral, sensory and motor function and movement in the kidneys.

From the beauty point of view it definitely reduces dark rings under the eyes or sunken or puffy look around the eyes.
Indications for Nasal medication - Headache, migraine, stiffness in head, neck, shoulders, lock-jaw, dental pain, nasal pain, eye pain, sinusitis, facial paralysis, epilepsy,

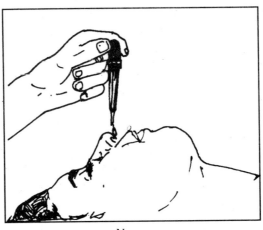
Nasya

sleeplessness, loss of speech in short any diseases of nose, eye, ear and throat. Medicines used for this purpose is -oils, pastes, powders, plant juices, decoctions, infusions also smoke.

Contra indications for *Nasya*
Pregnancy, menstruation, after hot bath, after eating or meal, after sexual interaction, after drinking alcohol.

Types of *Nasya*
Shodhana - or cleansing *nasya* - purifying
Shamana - Pacifying *nasya* - Reduces doshas
Brihana - Tonification - for nourishing

Technique
i) Pre procedure- Apply suitable oil on face, forehead, shoulder and nasal region and give steam or dry fomentation to this region. Allow patient to lie down, and ask him to raise his head in such a way that the nose should be directed upwards towards ceiling.
ii) Main procedure- Put 4 to 8 drops of warm oil, juice or

decoction in right nostril. Close the left nostril and ask the patient to inhale the same. Repeat this with left nostril.

iii) Post procedure - allow the patient to remain in this position for 10 seconds and then ask him to lie on the bed with normal position. If the oil or medicine comes in the throat, he can swallow the same or spit it out.

Pradhamana Nasya

It is a specific type of *nasya*, which is used mainly for purification purpose. A special apperatus is available for this purpose, which has main container with the nossel and the rubber bulb attatched to the same. Powder or the liquid medicine is filled in the main container. Then the nossel is put into the nostril after preliminary procedure and the proper position. Then the rubber buld is pressed in such a way that approximately 125 mgm. Powder is administered in the nostril. The medicines used for this purpose are usually of hot potency and of penetrating quality. Therefore there the nasal secretions will start immediately. After proper purification, as the patient to take rest.

Vapor Nasya

Leaves of medicine or decoction is kept on boiling. Patient is advised to cover his face and head with a towel and inhale the vapor.

Benefits

Elimination of vitiated doshas from nose. Lightness in head and body, good sleep, proper functioning of sense organs and mind, relief of symptoms for which nasya is done.

It is effective for treating disease above the region of clavicle. Many diseases of eye, ear, neck, head, thoat can be treated with this method. This should be given as supportive treatment

101

along with the massage treatement in this region.

6. FEET

Padabhyanga

Foot massage is highly praised in Ayurveda. Before going to bed it is very useful to have a massage over the soles of the feet. Every day foot massage preserves man from diseases of eyes and other organs and brings peace, prosperity and good luck. According to ancient Ayurvedic scriptures diseases do

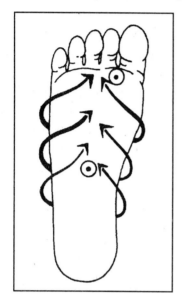 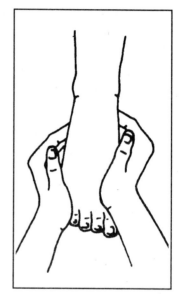

Padabhyanga

not go near one who massages his feet before sleeping just as snakes do not approach eagles. One should carry out foot massage for treating dryness, numbness, roughness, fatigue and lack of sensation and cracking in the soles of feet. It promotes strength for walking and running and gives sturdiness to the limbs.

102

A beneficial description of effects of foot massage is written in *Vagbhata*. According to him there are four important nerves in the sole of feet which are connected to the head. Because of heat, friction and excessive pressure on the feet, these nerves get affected as a result of which eyesight of a person gets reduced. But after giving massage to the soles a person never suffers from eye diseases. Also one must note important basic principle, that feet (*karmendriya*) and eye (*dnyanendriya*) both are related with element of fire. Hence although they are far apart from each other they are interconnected with each other. Hence it advisable to apply castor oil to the sole and then massage the feet with the bottom of copper vessel. This is extremely beneficial in case of burning of eyes due to excessive walking in Sun or for those who are masseures.

A simple mustard oil massage prevents cold weather cracking and peeling of skin. It reduces and eliminates infections caused by fungus and bacteria also. When full bath or shower is not possible simply bathing feet with hot or cold water produces freshness in the whole body.

Benefits of foot massage
Increased foot strength, ability to stand continuously for long periods. One can avoid hardness, stiffness, roughness, tiredness and insensibility to touch. It is also beneficial for treating cracks in the sole and varicose veins and for improvement in eyesight. After proper foot massage, person gets better sleep.

The science of Reflexology states that the sole of feet has connections with various organs of the body. Hence proper foot massage at respective site on the foot with specific oils prevents and cures various diseases. According to this science, various organs like heart, lungs, kidney, brain, intestines all can be stimulated by feet massage. Above all a massage helps a person to have sound sleep at night.

7. NAILS

The fingernails are the byproduct (*mala*) of the *asthi dhatu* (bones). Each tissue is inter-related as they nourish each other in a sequential fashion. The condition of nails is not only influenced by the blood quality but also by electro-magnetic

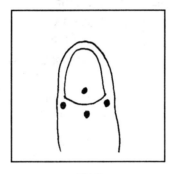

Nail

energy that flows through the body in the system of meridians. Thumbnail is an indicator for brain. Index finger nail is indicator for lungs and colon. Middle finger for small intestine, Ring finger for kidney and little finger for the heart.

Healthy nails are pinkish in color, smooth and evenly shaped. The actual shape and consistency varies with which dosha is dominant.

Vata type nails tends to be most irregular in shape and prone to being pale and brittle.

Pitta nails are an even oval shape, soft, flexible and pink.

Kapha nails are square, thick and strong.

104

White spots on nails shows calcium and zinc deficiency. Bitten nails show nervousness, mineral deficiency., Hang nails show lack of proteins, vitamins. Brittle nails show low iron or Vit. A. Split nails show low *agni* in stomach. Yellowish nails show liver imbalance. Bluish nails show lung and heart imbalance. Pale nails show poor blood circulation, anemia.

Old people always complain about crack nails. Also people wearing shoes regularly also complain crack nails or turned nails and pain in nail beds.

The diet should be rich in proteins and nail building minerals such as sulfur, iron calcium and silica as well as vitamins D and E. Regular massage to nails and nail beds, and nail surrounded area is very important for nail beauty. On a daily basis - dip fingers in warm water. Use very soft nail brush for cleaning nails and fingers. Then putting a drop of sesame oil on nail and nail base do self massage very gently to nail beds and nails.

Apply herbal pastes containing *Triphala, Karanj* and *neem* with aloe gel, once in a week to nails and nail base for 20 minutes and then wash with warm water and lemon juice. This is helpful for nourishment of nails. It gives normal appearance and shine to nails.

8. VERTEBRAL COLUMN

Vertebral column is a main seat of *avalambak Kapha*, spinal cord, *asthi* and *majja dhatu*. There are 24 vertebras 7 - cervical, 12-thorasic and 5-lumber region. Having three natural curves, the vertebras are connected to each other by muscles, ligaments and joints. There are 22 discs between these vertebras & nerves pass through the openings in the vertebras.

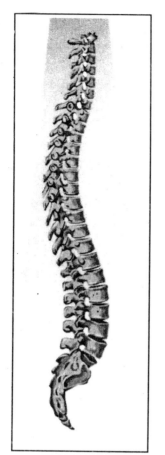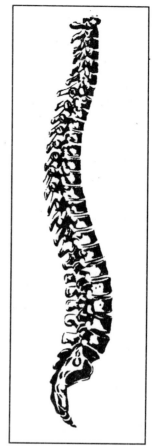

Vertebral Column

If a spine is properly aligned and strong, the vital life force will flow in the body for longer duration. If the spine is in right shape the man will think right, act right and live an energetic life. At the time of massage, masseur must learn how to put all vertebrae in proper alignment. Another important thing is the role of the spinal fluid in maintaining the health, vigor, vitality and virility. Massage of the spine can cure nervous and all psychic disorders.

The psychic centers work through ductless glands. By massaging the spine a massagist can slowly bring about a change in the body and release from tension. Massage without oil and without pressure is not effective on the spine. Before starting massage oil is applied all over the spinal cord, by using friction, giving alternate pressure by by two thumbs. Massage is done using kneading, tamping. Twisting of the spine to the right and left is the best exercise for the spinal cord. This increases circulation of spinal fluid.

Benefits
Stiffnes and back pain gets relieved.
Nervous system works properly.
Tension in mind also gets released.

1.*Kundalini* massage
The human spine is a seat of miracles. Yoga and Tantra - the science that deals with evolution of human consciousness are full of the description of the mysterious powers. '*Kundalini*' the serpent power that operates through spine lies at the base of the vertebral column. The spine is a seat of all chakras, psychic centers except the sixth *chakra*. The central nervous system and autonomous nervous system also works through spine.

Kundalini massage is very ancient art of massage. Although we do not find any direct reference to this special type of massage in any yoga textbooks or in connection with *Kundalini yoga*, this massage is parctised in many yoga schools in India. *Kundalini* is the seed energy of the subtle body. It resides at the base of the vertebral column, in the root *chakra. Kundalini* contains within itself all the powder of consciousness.

Dr. David Frawley in his book 'From the river of heaven' has explained that, kundalini can be recognised as intense power of devotion or attention. This is related with Yoga of devotion and Yoga of knowledge. In neither of these two systems of Yoga is any special method for awakening the *kundalini* is required. It is usually suppliment these two Yogas, in the absence of their full power, that methods to arouse the *kundalini* may be used. The proper awakening of *kundalini* is

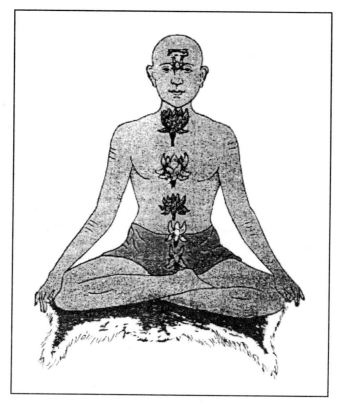

The six Chakras

108

through Divine grace. If artificial methods like *kundalini* massage or willful, forced or egoistic practises are used there can be possible side effects. Hence it is advisable that *kundalini* massage must be done under supervision and with proper care. This does not mean that any effort on our part is not useful but that our effort must be to attune ourselves to the grace. The premature arousing of *kundalini* can burn up nervous system and can limit or prevent our spiritual growth permentaly.

The arousing of the *kundalini* is usually brought about through coordination of posture, massage, breath and mantra. For *kundalini* massage one can use proper medicated oil. Ask the patient to lie on the abdomen. Start the massage at the bottom of the spine and go upwards up to the cervical spine. There is another method in which instead of using only one oil for the entire massage, masseur can use different oils at different *chakras*.

2. Lymph drainage massage
Massage works directly with the three circulatory systems of the body simultaneously
Blood vascular system
Nervous system
Lymphatic system

The lymphatic system is the one, which is most directly involved in massage. The lymphatic system works through ducts, nodes and passages. This system is supplementary system to the blood vascular system. It runs side by side with the blood circulatory system and through osmosis gets mixed with blood and supplied to whole body. The lymphatic system assists blood circulation by draining excess fluids from the

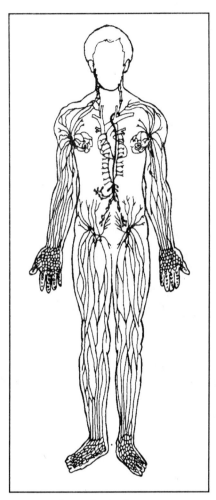

Lymphatic System

blood streams easing the workload of heart, lymphatic system offers an alternative route for the return of tissue fluid to the blood stream. Masseur must remember that the lymph nodes which produce lymphatic fluid are located underneath all the joints of the body and by rubbing and applying circular movement one can stimulated these lymph nodes by massage.

Also pressure, fomentation and deep breathing exercises can stimulate the system. By using oil massage (rubbing) cleanses and vitalizes the body. So massage is ideal for older people whose muscles and tendons are week.

Increasing lymph flow reduces blood pressure this is one of the reasons for giving massage for blood pressure patients. Regular massage relaxes the system and aids digestion by maintaining a proper balance and proper circulation of gases.

The lymphatic massage may be particularly useful when employed in a preventive health care system for the layman. Lymphatic massage causes a number of subjective changes in mood. It is a painless massage. It is also associated with marmas (Vital points).

The ancient Indians felt that the benefits of massage were medicated by increasing the flow of lymph in lymph vessels and ascribed to lymph the properties of increasing viscosity, nourishment, solidarity, sexual stamina etc.

Massage for relaxation

For relaxation massage should be done very gentle. In the cases of mental and physical strain, anxiety, worries, insomnia, weakness of muscles, cramps also in old age massage is done very gently. Massage of spine, shoulder, leg and hands help in these cases.

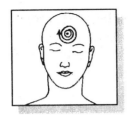

11.
Marma Massage

All vital points are very sensitive areas. Hence massage at these vital points should be done very carefully, by using thumb. (However knuckle, wrist, palm and heel of the foot are also used in specific therapy). By stimulating marma points by massage one can bring healing effects to specific area of mind body system. These points were also used for stimulating internal organs and system of the body.

The movement should be clock-wise, when stimulation of internal organs or channels or tissues has to be done. (Imagine putting the clock on the body of the patient and then follow

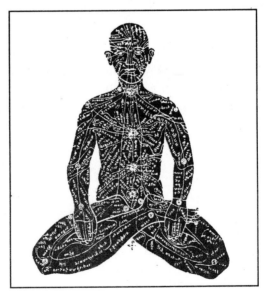

the movement of the clock). When aggravated doshas are to be alleviated or the excess tissue growth is to be reduced, the massage should be done anti clock-wise. At least 3 to 5 minutes massage every day for 2 times, should be done. One can use heavy oils or aromatic oils for this massage. It has been observed that with this massage one can control internal channels and organs and can treat doshas also.

For balancing doshas, following oils can be used.
Vata - Sesame, olive, almond.
 Basil, cedarwood, cinnamon, clove, geranium, jasmine, lavender, myrrh, musk, orange, and sage.
Pitta - Coconut, sunflower, sandalwood
 Camomile, cinnamon, gardenia, honeysuckle, lotus,

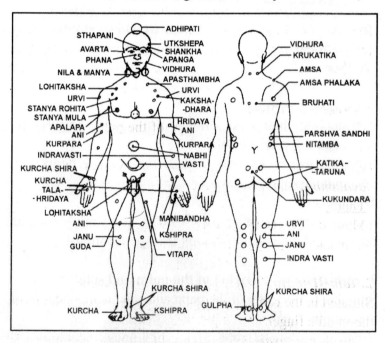

Marma Points

113

mint, rose and saffron.

Kapha - Mustard, sesame, corn, jojoba. Basil, camphor, clove,
eucalyptus, frankincense, juniper,
Lemon, marjoram, musk, myrrh, peppermint, rosemary
and sage.

Finger units (*anguli*) relative to each individual measure *Marma* points. Their size is measured by finger, inches and their location is determined by them. However they are different from acupuncture points.

There are 107 *marma* points. However for therapy we have explained only 21 important *marma* points in this chapter. Those who are interested in further studies of this science should read the book '*Marma* Therapy' written by Prof. Ranade, Dr. Lele and Dr. David Frawley, Published by International Academy of Ayurveda, Karve Road, Pune 411,004

1. *Kshipra* - (Quick)

Between thumb and index finger of the palm and great toe and index finger of the sole.

Controls *rasavaha* and *pranavaha srotas*, heart and *avalambaka* kapha,

Therapy

Massage- One can use powder of vacha, heavy oils like vacha oil, mustard oil, and amruta oil (Tinospora cordifolia).

2. *Tala-Hridaya* - (Heart of the palm and sole)

Situated in the center of the palm and sole facing the root of the middle finger.

Controls *pranavaha* srotas, Heart and Lungs, respiration and *avalambaka* Kapha.

114

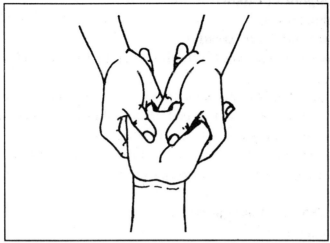

Tala-Hridaya

<u>Therapy</u>
Massage -use *Narayan* oil.

3. *Kurcha* - (A knot or bundle of the muscles at the base of the thumb) -
Situated 1 inch distal from the wrist joint at the root of the thumb, above *kshipra marma*. And also in the sole.
Controls *alochaka* Pittà
<u>Therapy</u>
Massage -massage with sandalwood oil, or *shatadhauta ghrita* - ghee washed in water for 100 times and aromatic oils like rose and lotus are useful.

4. *Indra basti* - ('Indra's bladder'- mid fore arm and mid calf region)-
Controls *annavaha*, *agni* and small intestine.
<u>Therapy</u>
Massage - For stimulation of agni use of *mahamasha* oil is good.

115

5, *Kurpara* - (Elbow)

In cubital fossa.

Controls *raktavaha srotas*.

Marma on rt. controls Liver, *Marma* on Lt. Controls spleen.

Therapy

Massage- For liver diseases massage should be done on the right *kurpara marma*. Use padmakadi oil or manjisthadi oil or aromatic oils like rosemary are good.

For diseases of spleen left *kurpara marma* should be massaged with oil of ginger (zingiber officinalis).

6. *Gulpha* -   (Ankle joint)

Ankle joint.

Controls *medovaha, asthivaha*, and *shukravaha* srotas.

Therapy

Massage -use ashwagandha oil, triphaladi sahasrayoga oil for females and nutmeg (myristica fragrans) for males

7. *Janu* - (Knee)

On the Knee Joint.

Right *marma* controlls liver, Left marma controlls spleen

Therapy

Massage- For improving function of liver massage on the right marma with nalapamaradi oil and for improving spleen massage on the left *marma* with bhringamalakadi oil.

8. *Vitap* -   (The perinium) - One inch lateral to the syphysis pubis.

Controls *shukravaha srotas*.

Therapy

Massage - For controlling *shukravaha srotas*, it is advisable to massage with mashataila, kumkumadi oil.

9. *Guda* - (Anus)

Controls 1 *chakra- muladhara* and channels of urinary, reproduction, menstrual as well as testes and ovaries.

<u>Therapy</u>

Massage - For improving function of emmenagouge, use saffron (crocus sativus) or oil of myrrrh. For increasing sexual function, use musk or honeysuckle. It is also advisable to use agaru oil (aquillaria agallocha) as rejuvenative massage in men.

For controlling obesity, use asana-bilwadi oil for massage.

10. *Basti* - (Bladder)

Above and behind symphisis pubis.

Controls *mamsavaha srotas* and *apana Vata*.

<u>Therapy</u>

Massage- For controlling Vata, use dashamuladi oil, sesame oil or narayan oil.

11. *Nabhi* -(Umbilicus)

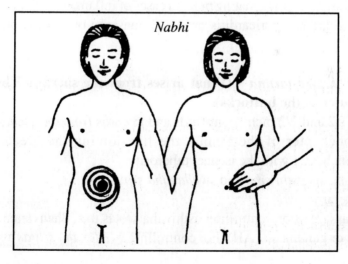

Nabhi

Controls 3-rd *chakra- manipura*, Channels of *annavaha* and *raktavaha*.

Pancreas, *agni*- Solar plexus, *pachaka, ranjaka Pitta; samana Vata*.

Therapy

Massage - For increasing digestion use oil of ginger or fennel. Using massage of nabhighruta (ghee+rock salt+ camphor) to relieve gas in children is very effective. For this pour sufficient quantity of this ghee in umbilicus and then insert one finger in it. Then carry out pinching type of massage. There will be instant relief of pain and gas accumulated in intestines.

12. *Hridaya* (Heart)

Controls *rasavaha srotas, sadhaka Pitta, vyana* and *prana Vata, Ojus, avalambaka Kapha* and 4 th *chakra* or *anahata*.

Therapy

Hrid basti -is very effective for controlling aggravated Vata, in cases of irregular heartbeats, arrhythmia, angina pectoris etc.

Massage - for alleviating pitta, in cases of inflamatory diseases of heart 'like pericarditis or S.B.E. massage of sandalwood oil.

13. *Katika-taruna* - (What arises from the sacrum. The center of the buttocks)

It is 2 and 1/2 inch downwards and inwards from the greater tronchanter of the Femur, the line joining the greater tronchanter with the ischael tuberosity.

Controls *asthivaha* and *swedavaha srotas*.

Therapy

Massage- For controlling asthivaha srotas use, dhanvantara oil or gandha oil (AH). For controlling *swedavaha srotas* use

118

kakolyadi oil for massage.

14. *Kukundara* - (Marking on the loins on either side of posterior superior Iliac sine)
On both post. Superior iliac spine notches.
Controls *raktavaha* - formation of blood.
Ischaeum bone. (No joint structure)
Therapy
Massage - For stimulating *raktavaha srotas* use, manjishthadi oil or kottamchukadi oil (calamus + garlic+ galangal).

15. *Bruhati* - (The large or the broad region of the back)
Three inches above the Inferior angle of the scapula in the middle border, at the triangular space.
Controls 4 th *chakra- anahata* and *rasavaha srotas.*
Therapy
Massage-For improving the functions of *rasavaha srotas*, use rasataila (bala+meat) or himasagara oil (asperagus+manjishtha -rubia cordifolia- + kushmanda) (BR). For *annavaha srotas* aromatic oil of fennel (foeniculum vulgare) is indicated.

16. *Amsa* - (The shoulder)
Between the neck and arms, on the trapezius muscle. 1/2 inch lateral to 5 th Cervical vertebra.
Controls 5 th *chakra, Vishudha. Bhrajaka* Pitta, *Udana* Vata and Brain
Therapy
Massage- Controls 5 th *chakra (vishudha)*, For controlling bhrajaka pitta oils of jasmin and kewada are best.

17. *Apanga* - (The outer corner of the eye)
At the outer angle of eye. Lateral side of orbital fossa.

Controls Sense organ of sight.

Therapy

Massage- For treating sense organ of sight, use of triphala oil or aromatic oil of vetiver(vetivera zizanoides) is advised.

18. *Shankha* - ('Conch' the temple)

In between the tragus of the ear and the lateral corner of the eye.

Controls sense organs of touch and Vata in large Intestine.

Therapy

Massage - For treating any problems of sense organ of touch (skin) use ashwagandha oil.

19. *Adhipati* - (The lord of all) Posterior Frontalle. Top of the cranium.

Controls 7 th *chakra- sahasrara* and *majjavaha srotas, prana Vata, tarpaka Kapha* and *sadhaka Pitta.*

Therapy

After birth, the anterior fontanel is wide open. Due to incomplete ossification, the top portion of the skull is only covered by thin skin. For quick healing it is therefore advisable to apply sesame oil.

Pichu dharana - keeping gauze diped in medicated oils like dhanvantara is useful for treating Vata disorders.

Abhyanga- For treating sadhaka pitta disorders in brain, use oil of brahmi

for treating disorders of Prana, use oil of dhanvantara, For treating disorders of tarpaka kapha use oil of -cedarwood.

20. *Sthapani* - (That gives support)

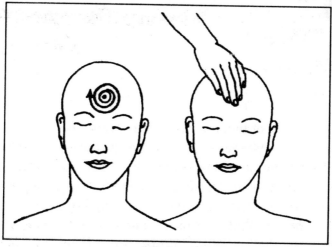

Sthapani

In between the eyebrows. Position of third eye.
Controls 6 th *chakra- ajnya* and *prana*
<u>Therapy</u>
Shirodhara - For treating disorders of 6 th *chakra (ajnya)* and prana Vata, pouring slow drip of dhanvantara oil on this *marma* is very useful.

21. *Simanta* - (The sumit, the skull and the surrounding joints)
coronal, sagital and lambdoid sutures in the skull.
Controls *majjavaha, rasavaha* and *raktavaha srotas.*
<u>Therapy</u>
Abhyanga- application of medicated oils like dhanvantara, bhrungaraja to the *marma* is useful for alleviation of doshas.
Keeping *pichu* - cotton dipped in medicated oil- at the point is also useful.
Soon after the delivery, sesame oil should be applied to this *marma* for controlling Vata.

121

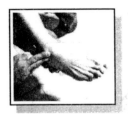

12.
Massage for specific Diseases

1. Arthritis

Inflammation of the joints is called arthritis. It can be acute or chronic. In Ayurveda it is commonly known as Sandhivata. Sandhi means joint and vitiation of Vata is usually the prominent factor in this disease. Acute arthritis may result due to trauma, infections, gout, or hemophilia. Similarly it can be due to toxins commonly known as ama. When this toxin mixes with a vitiated dosha, it can cause amavata or rheumatic arthritis. Chronic arthritis can also be due to different infections like tuberculosis and collagen as well as degenerative disorders. Immunological disorders and vitiation of doshas are many times responsible for chronic arthritis.

a. Traumatic Arthritis

Vata vitiation is the predominant factor in the pathogenesis. If there are no visible injuries on the skin, then external application of curcuma amada with lime is beneficial.
Massage -Apply Vishgarbha oil and then carry out the fomentation of the affected joint.

b. Rheumatic Arthritis

In Ayurveda this is called as *amavata*. A low digestive fire produces *ama* or toxins in the digestive tract, which then circulates the entire body from the heart and blood vessels causing a fever, heart disorders, and joint problems. The disease starts in the stomach, manifests in the joints and the heart, and then spreads at the Kapha dosha sites in the body.

Symptoms

The main symptom of this disease is a fleeting type of pain in the big joints. The inflammation and pain shifts from joint to joint very rapidly. In the acute stage, the big joints are inflamed on a given day and then absolutely normal the next day when some other joint becomes affected.

When the heart gets involved usually the mitral valve is affected and there is either stenosis or regurgitation type deformity. Hence it is said that this disease "bites the joints and leaks the heart." Therefore when *ama* is present in the digestive system, one should never carry out excessive exercise. Also at this stage vigorous massage to the inflamed joints is contrandicated. Otherwise *ama* spreads throughout the entire body and can cause serious complications.

Treatment

To destroy *ama*, fasting should be carried out in the acute stage. The swollen joints should be fomented by dry heat either by electrical pads or by using hot sand or infrared lamp. One teaspoon of castor oil should be taken internally with garlic tea, which will detoxify ama in 3-4 days.

Ama stage

In this stage, the joints are inflamed, swollen, and very painful. Application of prasarani oil (BP) helps to relieve severe pain in this acute condition.

Until the *ama* is detoxified, the patient should take only warm vegetable soup. Whenever the patient is thirsty, he should

123

drink warm water or herbal tea.

Nirama stage
In this stage the swelling of the joints disappears but they are still very much painful. When *ama* gets detoxified, this 'no *ama*' stage is present.

Massage
Use sahacharadi oil, rasona oil or saindhavadi oil for massage. During this stage patient can take light diet, which will not disturb digestive fire. Soup of white meat, basmati rice, ghee, buttermilk or milk and plenty of fruit juice can be taken with green vegetables.

c. Rheumatoid Arthritis

Vitiated Vata affects the joints and produces this disease. This is also known as *'Sandhigata Vata'*. The small and large affected joints are painful and swollen. If it is not treated properly, after chronic stage, deformity may develop in affected joints. People after 40 are affected most often. It is a systemic connective tissue disorder affecting joints, hence muscle wasting, and inflammation of muscles around the joint is very common.

Symptoms
In typical Vata type, the pain is throbbing, migrating, and cutting. It is relieved by fomentation. Deformity is more likely to take place. Other symptoms of Vata aggravation like constipation, gas, nervousness, and insomnia are common. Pitta type Joints are more inflamed, red, hot to touch accompanied with fever, thirst and irritability. Pain increases by fomentation. In the Kapha type, there is more swelling

and edema around the joints, and the pain is dull aching type, which is relieved by fomentation.

Treatment
Vata type- affected joints should be massaged with sahacharadi oil and then fomentation with medicated vapor of herbs like basil.
Pitta type- Massage with kottamchukadi oil. A preparation called as chandanbalalakshadi oil, is alos useful in this condition.
Kapha type- For massage, apply oil is indicated. If the pain and swelling is too much, dry fomentation by infrared lamp or heated sandbag is beneficial.

d. Osteo Arthritis

This is also called as *Asthigata Vata*. This is the disease that occurs in people usually above 50 years. Affected joints are painful, patient also suffers from other symptoms of Vata vitiation like loss of sleep, weakness, and loss of strength in the muscles.

Treatment
Vata type-
Massage the joints with narayan oil, bala oil, or dhanvantari oil is very effective. When these oils are not available, use simple sesame oil, or one can cook available anti-arthritic herbs with sesame oil for external massage.
Pitta type- massage with nimb amrutadi oil with cold ice packs to the joints is useful.
Kapha type-
Massage with vishagarbha oil helps to loosen joints, detoxify the ama and improve the affected joint function. For this

purpose prasarini oil is the best.

Diet
Proper nutritive food with Vitamin A and D should be given. Natural calcium is available in many dairy products like cheese, milk, butter, and ghee. These should be taken with ghee and plenty of green vegetables.

f. Gout

According to Ayurveda, vitiated Vata and vitiated blood (rakta) causes this disease. Hence it is called as *Vatarakta*. Increased blood uric acid levels are also responsible for this disease.

Symptoms
Usually the disease starts from the inflammation of the big toe of the foot or the thumb of the hand. After this the other big or small joints in the body are affected. The disease originates in the circulatory system, gets localized into joints, and spreads throughout the body. The swollen joints are very painful, tender, inflamed, red, and warm to touch. High degree fever is usually present in acute stage. Many times skin rashes and allergic symptoms are also present with severe itching or change in the color of the skin. Excessive sweating or no sweating and severe pain in bones and muscles may be present.

Treatment
Purification by medicated purgation or blood letting according to the condition and stage of the disease is advised. Three specific herbs are used: tinospora cordifolia, kokilaksha (astercantha longifolia) and suranjana -(colchium luteum).

Massage
Apply lightly the oil prepared from guduchi or pinda taila should be applied to the swollen joints. In this condition, avoid deep massage. Internally, medicated ghee with guduchi is indicated. A simple combination of 500 mgm; each of guggulu with guduchi or colchium twice a day for 1 month, is very useful.

Technique
depending on the joint involved the massuer should be given free choice to carry out first circular massage aroung the joints. Later on he can proceed with petrissage combined with kneading and deep friction.

2. Backache

Although pain anywhere in the back is known as backache, usually it is connected to the vertebral column or the attached muscles. Backache is very common after 40 both in males and females.

Causative Factors
Various diseases of the vertebral column, spinal cord diseases, and meninges, fibrosis, lumbago, slipped disk, and other diseases of the abdominal and pelvic organs. Lack of calcium after delivery, obesity, tubercular infections, fractures, and tumors can also be responsible. In modern days however, defective posture, stress, and incorrect use of the back in lifting are the primary causes.

Treatment
Vata vitiation, bone weakness, and muscle weakness are the major factors to consider when providing treatment.

Massage

use mahamasha oil. Then mild fomentation or warm tub bath should be taken.

Technique

before starting the treatment, make sure that the patient soes not suffer from 'slipped disc'. The back muscles are very strong, hence the masseur will have to work deep and with lot of pressure on these muscles as well as the vertebras. It is advisable to start the treatment with effleurage over the lumber muscles. Then give light strokes so that the muscles will relax properly. Later on carry out petrissage and firm kneading type of massage. Lastly tapotment strokes should be carried out.

Since this is Vata disorder, Panchakarma procedure like alternate cleansing enema and oil enema is beneficial. For enema, 60 to 70 ml. of sesame oil should be used and it should be given preferably in the evening. Courses of alternate medicated enema 7, 10, or 15 should be given.

3. Cervical Spondilytis

Spondilon means vertebra. When there is inflammation in the ligaments and muscles surrounding the vertebras, this disorder is caused. This is high Vata and Pitta disorder.

Causative factors

As the age increases, there is natural tendency of wear and tear of the vertebras. When they becomes weak, they are afflicted by inflammation. Similar causes like trauma, disorder due to constant shocks by heavy equipment or bad road surface, incorrect posture like bending the neck while working at a computer, typing, writing, reading is also responsible for this problem.

Symptoms

Most commonly cervical vertebras are affected. There is pain in the neck that may radiate towards hands and fingers. Pain may be at the back near scapular region. Tingling and numbness to the hands is very common. Vertigo after bending neck may be present.

Treatment

It is useful to try the following mixture for three weeks: 2 teaspoons Castor oil, 2 teaspoons fresh juice of ginger, 1/4 teaspoon lemon juice, and 1 teaspoon ghee taken on empty stomach early in the morning. It is most important is to observe the correct posture while writing, typing, etc. Forward bending of the neck should be avoided. While sleeping care should be taken that pillow is not too thick, because larger the pillow, the neck remains more in the forward bending position which increases the problem.

Massage

The best oil is prabhanjana vimardana. It should be followed by nadi sweda fomentation with the mixture of water and few drops of eucalyptus oil or leaves of vitex negundo.

Technique

The neck contains many vital arteries and veins, which are connected to the brain. Therefore lot of caution must be taken while massaging the fornt portion of the neck. Undue pressure on carotids can cause serious trouble in the heart and other circulatory disturbances.

The back portion of the neck has cervical vertebras and various muscles and ligaments attatched to it. The massuer should massage these muscles from above downward direction.

4. Headache

Pain anywhere is always due to Vata vitiation. However, Pitta and Kapha can be associated with Vata for causing headaches. In Ayurveda headache is classified under the term "*Shiro roga.*" Ayurveda describes 11 types of headaches, and other diseases in which headache is the prominent symptom. There are two main causes of headaches: intracranial and extracranial.

Intracranial causes
Trauma, vascular headache due to migraine, hypertension, vasodilator drugs, alcohol hangover, withdrawal of habit forming drugs, and coffee.

Extracranial causes
includes trauma to soft tissues of scalp, bones, and sinuses. Reflex causes from eye, ear, and teeth also cause headache. Similarly stress and strain are responsible for tension headaches.

Symptoms
Vata type- is characterized by severe pain with anxiety, constipation, lack of sleep, and depression. It can be due to worry and strain.
Pitta type- headache is accompanied with a burning sensation, pain in the eyes, irritability, and photophobia. Migraine headache with nausea, vomiting, blurring of vision, and headache restricting to the half side of the head is usually Pitta type.
Kapha type- is dull aching pain with cold or heaviness in head.
Ardhavabhedaka- is typical migraine headache.
Suryavarta- In this type the intensity of headache increases

as the sun rises.

Shankhaka- In this type, headache is more prominent in the temporal region.

Anantavata- is due to vitiation of all doshas, this is a type in which the intensity is very severe.

<u>Treatment</u>
<u>Massage</u>
Vata type- Apply nimbpatradi oil to the head.
Pitta type - Massage the head with bhringamalakadi oil, padmakadi oil, himasagar oil or amalakyadi oil.
For all other types - application of dhanvantara oil, manjishthadi oil, triphaladi oil and durvadi oil is indicated.

<u>Technique</u>
The masseur should pour oil in his palm. Then he should dip his fingers in the oil and start massaging the scalp. For hair loss and other problems of hairs, he should should go along the lines of seemanta marma and pay proper attention to the adhipati marma.

5. Hemiplegia

Paralysis of one side of the body is known as hemiplegia. In Ayurveda it is called "*Pakshavadha.*" *Paksha* is, hand, foot, or one side of the body. *Vadha* is complete loss of function. It is classified under *vatavyadhi.* The term ardita denotes facial paralysis. All other diseases like paraplegia etc. are also grouped under the category of *vatavyadhi.*

<u>Causative factors</u>
It is Vata disorder involving the central nervous system and the muscular system. It can be due to cerebral tumor,

131

embolism, or hemorrhage. Other diseases of the brain and head trauma can produce hemiplegia, in which there may be paralysis on one side of the body with or without aphasia. Prana and vyana types of Vata are vitiated in this disorder.

Treatment

In case of complete paralysis of all the extremities, for first few days or weeks the patient is totally bedridden. In this case, all the necessary nursing care must be taken. A waterbed should be provided to avoid bed sores. Daily passive exercises must be given to avoid disuse atrophy of the extremities. In such condition, the patient is bound to become depressed. Those attending him should keep him engaged in reading or watching television.

Nasya- the main site of prana is the brain. Hence nasya or nasal instillation of ghee or cooling herbs juice is indicated.

Massage and sudation- Daily massage to the paralyzed limbs and whole body sudation is indicated. Abhyanga with simple sesame oil, almond oil, or narayan oil, bala oil or dhanvantari oil or karpasasthyadi oil will improves the circulation in the muscles and also helps improve the muscular tone. For sudation herbs like vitex negundo, basil, camphor should be used.

Medicated enema- the main site of Vata is large intestine or colon, hence to control Vata vitiation, this is the treatment of choice. It is advisable to give alternate cleansing enema and oil enema. For cleansing type of enema use, decoction of ten roots, dashamoola, and its paste with little oil, ghee, honey and rock salt. For medicated oil enema, use simple sesame oil 60 to 70 cc. or use medicated oil like narayan or bala oil. A simple glycerin syringe can be used for giving this oil enema. Along with this treatment

Shiro basti and Shirodhara- treatments are also very much

useful.

6. Poliomylitis

In Ayurveda it has been described as *"Bala pakshvadha."* It is common acute viral infection affecting various parts of central nervous system.

Causative factors
It is a disease of children under the age of 5 years. However during epidemics, older children and adults can get affected. It is due to high Vata and Pitta affecting nervous and muscular system.

Symptoms
In the early stage (prodromal) there may be symptoms of respiratory and gastrointestinal disturbances like coryza, sore throat, cough, nausea, vomiting, diarrhea, and other symptoms like fever, headache and irritability. These symptoms are more aggravated in preparalytic stage. In Paralytic stage which starts between second and fifth day, lower limbs are frequently affected; rarely upper limb paralysis and respiratory disturbances are found. During this time, fever is still present.

Treatment
Massage - To pacify vitiated vata, external massage is the best treatment. It should be started only when the tenderness in muscles disappears.
Chandan bala lakshadi oil, narayan oil, mahanarayan oil or dhanvantari oil bala oil or ksheera bala oil should be gently massaged followed by warm bath. 100 times potentised ksheera bala oil can be used for internal consumption in dose of 5 drops twice a day.

Pizicchil or fomentation by pouring hot medicated oil by drip method on the body is useful. Navarakkizi is another treatment in which patient is massaged with rice bolus cooked in medicated milk.

Both treatments are often combined with alternate oil enema and cleansing enemas. According to the predominance of doshas, particular herbs are selected for cleansing enemas. Brihan basti or special tonifying enema is indicated which is a mixture of milk, meat soup, honey, ghee and decoction of tonifying herbs. This should be given by drip method very slowly. This type of enema has much beneficial effects for increasing the tone of the paralyzed muscles.

Diet

Anti Vata diet should be given. Plenty of dairies like milk, ghee should be given. Meat soup, basmati rice, plenty green vegetables should be advised.

7. Sciatica

Pain along the distribution of sciatic nerve, due to inflammation, is a typical disorder of Vata vitiation. Most often this is due to lumbar disc prolapse. It can be due to injury, trauma to the vertebral column, or to the nerve proper. Various tumors of the spinal cord, different diseases of vertebral column like arthritis, tuberculosis, spondylolithiasis, or cancer. Some disorders of the hip joint like fibrositis and some particular disorders of pelvis also causes this syndrome.

Symptoms

There is severe pain along the root of the sciatic nerve that may travel down the back of the leg to the knee. The patient has lot of difficulty while walking. If the pain is constant, insomnia may also be present.

Treatment

Herbs like ricinus communis, rasna, bala, ashwagandha, guggulu and dashmoola are useful. Cleansing enema of dashmoola decoction alternatively with oil enema is indicated. Kati basti - It is a special type of basti which has good results for this problem. It should be done on the back from where the sciatic nerve originates. It is useful to relieve the inflammation and pain. For Kati basti, ask the patient to lie on the abdomen. Prepare wheat flour dough and with that make two inch circular portions over the sciatic area on the back. These portions should be able to hold warm medicated oil without leaking. Pour the oil in this area and keep the flour dough portions there for 20 minures.

Massage

In *sama* conditions use vishagarbha or prassarani oil. In nirama conditions use Mahanarayana oil. The massage should be done along the line of sciatic nerve.

Massage - with vishgarbha oil, saindhavadi oil or prasarini oil is advised. Afterwards, fomentation with basil leaves mixed in water by bringing the medicated vapor through a tube at the site of pain is very useful.

8. Constipation

Bowel movements differ from individual to individual. They depend on the type of diet and the general activity of the person. However constipation can be defined as accumulation of toxins in the colon due to improper bowel movements.

Ideally, one should have easy bowel movement in early morning and the stool should float on the water. If the stool sinks, is sticky, or has a very bad smell, this indicates the

135

presence of ama or toxins in the colon.

Causative factors-

Developing the proper urge in the morning is very important. The modern lifestyle of getting up late in the morning and rushing to work does not allow this habit to develop, which can lead to constipation. All Vata constitution persons suffer from this problem.

The main cause is dietary, eating a late meal after sundown or eating food that is hard to digest and that produces toxins in the colon. Food without roughage, too much coffee and tea, eating dry substances like legumes, drinking too cold drinks and smoking contribute to constipation.

Symptoms

The tongue is the mirror of digestion. Usually the tongue has a slightly whitish coating when we get up from the bed. But after scraping of the tongue (a practice that should be done in addition to brushing the teeth every morning) this coating disappears.

Treatment

Acute constipation - For immediate relief, give 60 to 70 ml. of warm sesame oil enema. Massage the abdomen with sesame oil and carry out light fomentation of the abdomen. If it is not possible, apply glycerin suppository. If the tongue is white coated, it means that there are lot of toxins in the colon. Fasting, anti-ama diets, and herbs to detoxify should be given. When the digestion is improved, then give strong purgatives like senna, rhubarb, or castor oil.

Chronic constipation - Giving laxatives or purgatives cannot treat this, because constant use of purgatives creates dryness in the colon that in turn increases constipation.

Triphala can be given in dose of 1 to 3 gms; at night, with

warm water. Triphala also acts as a rejuvenating medicine in old age.

Abhayarishta is also a medicine of choice for this condition. 30 ml. twice day should be given for 1 month.

Massage

Regular massage with the help of preper oils is excellent treatment for chronic constipation. The patient should be massage on empty stomach after his bladder and bowel is empty. This should be followed by kneading movements which are light at first and then becoming deeper and firmer. Then he should start friction movements, beginning at the lower left side of the abdomen and moving upwards but with downwards pressure, in small circles.

Chronic constipation is many times due to lack of tone in the musculature of the abdominal muscles. This type of massage strengthens the muscles of the abdomen and brings good tone to the mucsulature of the coplon.

Diet

Correction of dietary habits is a must. It is advisable to take lot of green vegetables cooked or uncooked, plenty of fruits, with oily and bulk-forrning foods containing high amount of roughage or fiber. Food must be taken at proper time, irregular food habits cause constipation.

9.Maramus

It is also known as "Kwashiorkor," a disease affecting infants and young children.

Causative factors

It is high Vata and low digestive fire disorder leading to wasting. Usually it is due to insufficient diet or inability to eat properly due to local lesions of mouth and jaw. There may be impaired absorption due to bowel diseases, like sprue. Children having low birth weight, brain tumor, or mental retardation may contract this disease.

Symptoms

Edema, skin changes, impaired growth, and fatty liver characterize this. There is typical appearance of a "Pot belly" which gives a false impression of health or overnutrition. The child becomes apathetic, but irritable and has a weak cry. The disease has periods of exacerbation and remission. In acute stage, the child may suffer from diarrhoea and dysentery.

Treatment

Massage- the best treatment for improving digestive power is to give regular massage with Vata palliating oils like bala oil, ksheerabala oil, narayan oil, and dhanvantari oil (YR) every day and exposure to early morning sun for 15 minutes. It has been observed that children deprived of proper food for long time cannot start taking regular dietery substances. In such cases, it is advisible to give regular massage with cow's milk. This milk used for the purpose of massage, gets absorbed and is useful for nourishment.

10. Rickets

This is also a disease occurring in infancy and early childhood, due to deficiency of Vitamin D, affecting bones in the body. In Ayurveda it is called as "*Phakka*" and is Vata disease.

Symptoms

Marasmic children are seldom rachitic, but as soon as the infant begins to put on weight, rickets is likely to develop. Because it develops only when growth starts taking place and there is deficiency of Vitamin D and calcium. The infant with rickets is characteristically restless, cries frequently, and may perspire excessively. Muscles of abdomen and limbs become very weak without tone, with abdominal distention. Normal developmental activities like crawling, sitting are delayed and the eruption of teeth is prolonged. Various deformities in bones of skull and thorax develop.

Treatment

The bony deformity may become permanent if it is not treated in time. Therefore start the treatment as early as possible.

Massage - Give regular massage to baby with any of the following oils chandan bala lakshadi oil, dashapak baladi oil, ashwangadhadi oil, narayan oil and expose the child to early morning sun or to infra red light for 15 to 20 minutes.

11. Varicose veins

When the veins become distended and tortuous this condition is known as varicose veins. This is a major cosmetic problem in women who are working as dancers, actresses, waitereses in hotels etc.

Causative factors

Defective or weak valves associated with postural strain, which obstructs venous blood flow, cause them. Constipation, irregularity, and jobs with continuous standing are the main causes. Vata constitution people suffer most from this disorder. It can be due to pressure in the abdominal cavity such as pregnancy. In pregnancy, the varicosity is temporary. In early cases there are no complaints, and patient often consults the doctor for cosmetic purpose only. But when the varicosity increases, there is pain after standing and the affected leg feels heavy.

Treatment

It is important that patient should not wear tight clothes. Ask the patient to apply elastic bandages at particular part of the leg to prevent further development of varicosity. For women, wearing stockings helps the prevention. It is also advisable to raise the legs while sleeping at least for 1 to 2 hours every day.

Massage

Never carry out kneading type of massge or never put pressure on the varicose veins.

Use warm sesame oil, narayan oil, or bala oil in the upward direction from foot to groin, twice a day. After massage keep the leg in warm water for fomentation. This will strengthen the valves in the veins and the condition will improve. Tab.shatavari and tab.ashwagandha 500 mgm; twice a day, with ashwagandharishta 15·ml. 3 times a day for 1 month is useful.

12. Obesity

Obesity is the most common metabolic disorder and is one of the oldest documented diseases. In Ayurveda as early as 1500 BC Charaka Samhita has described this disorder under the title "Medoroga" or diseased state of fat metabolism. According to Charaka, the great Ayurvedic physician, an individual whose increased adipose and muscle tissue makes his hips, abdomen, and breasts pendulous and whose vitality is much less than his body size is obese.

Causative factors

Simple obesity is due to alimentary factors like overeating heavy, sweet, oily foods. Lack of exercise and hereditary predisposition. It can be due to other disorders of pituitary, thyroid, adrenals, gonads, pancreas, and hypothalamus.

Symptoms

Apart from the signs described above, *Charaka* has described that such person has reduction of longevity, premature aging, unpleasant odor, excessive sweating, dyspnoea on mild exertion, excessive hunger and thirst, weakness, loss of vitality, loss of sexual power, and mental confusion.

Treatment

To increase the tissue fire of fatty tissue, herbs like guggulu, carthamus tinctoris, careya arborea, and shilajatu are used. Formation of ama is treated by toxin burning herbs like trikatu and catechu. Aggravation of Vata is treated by medicated enemas of cleansing type. Channel blocking is treated by fat reducing - lekhana - herbs, which have scraping action to open channels like chitraka and barbery. Externally the same herbs are used for massage with acorus calamus.

Regular active exercise every day until there is perspiration on the temple and axila is a must. It can be in the form of cycling, swimming, jogging, running, or outdoor activities. Massage- Only udvartana type of massage using dry and hot powders of calamus- vacha or satala etc. should be used. The massage must be very deep and little pain producing. Only this massage will be able to move the fatty tissue from the thighs, buttocks and other regions.

Diet

Avoid all fried heavy foods, chocolates, sweets, butter, cheese, paneer, red meat, as well as cold drinks and preserved foods. Light diet is recommended to provide only the necessary energy.

13.Massage for sportsmen

Professional sportsmen value massage very highly not because it works on several levels. Used before exercise it can prepare the body for the increased activity not only by warming and loosening the muscles and joints but increasing their flexibility and helping to prevent cramps and injury. It also stimulates the system both physically and mentally.

This is a key to improve performance. After an exercise session massage speeds up the elimination of waste products by stimulating the lymphatic system. Massage is done for longer periods to joints than the muscles. (see sports massage oil in chapter 14)

Strain and sprain

Burning sensation under the skin indicates that muscle fibers or ligaments have been strained- stretched beyond their natural limit. A routine of pre-exercise massage and limbering will help to prevent strains. Gently massaging the affected area help speedy recovery.

Sprains are more serious and are caused by violent wrenching of joints most commonly ankles, wrist or knee. The surrounding muscles, ligaments and tendons may also be damaged and affected area may be swollen or painful.

Applying ice pack for 15 to 20 minutes. Give gentle massage to affected area. The best oils for massage in this condition are prasarani and vishagarbha oil. Similarly product like myostal liniment is also very much useful in this condition.

Cramps

Frequent cramps may indicate generally poor circulation. Massage will increase the blood circulation to alleviate the pain.

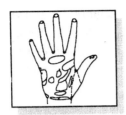

13.
Other healing systems related to massage

1. TCM - Acupressure

Ayurveda and Chinese are probably the two oldest healing system still practised all over the world. Being Oriental, both systems believe in maintaining the equilibrium of energies in

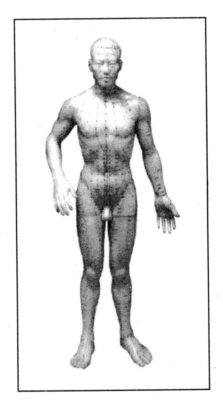

the body and talk about the importance of elements.

Traditional Chinese Medicine talks about yin and yang energies and tries to maintain their equilibrium with herbs, diet, acupuncture and acupressure. The system believes that the energy flows through certain meridians and the blockage can cause disturbance or diseases in the body. To relieve this blockage acupuncture and acupressure is helpful.

2. Reflexology

It is said that early Egyptian and Chinese civilizations were practising this science which was sometimes called as ' Zone Therapy'. The basis of this technique is that reflex zones mapped out on the feet and hands are related to different areas of the body.

Reflexology known today is based largly on the work done by Dr. William Fitzgerald and Eunice Ingham.This science states that our hands and feet have specific areas, which are linked to all internal organs. These organs can be stimulated for health and therapeutic purposes through the massage and manipulations from the areas of the hands and feet.

It is based on the principle that the body can be divided into ten vertical zones, each corresponding to an area of the foot, so that the feet are in effect a map of the body.

A sensitive area of the foot indicates a problem in the corresponding organ of the body and by working on the appropriate painful spot, the problem can be solved.

Use of proper oils and manipulations through these areas can bring about-

1. Reduction of stress and strain
2. Stimulation of different organs, systems and glands, for

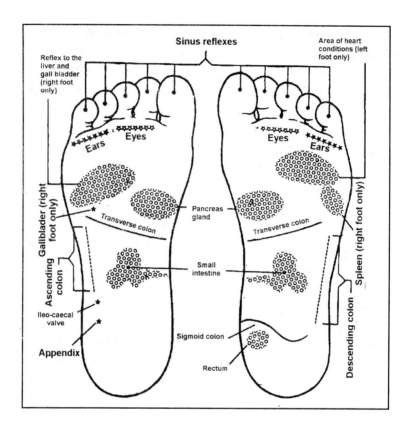

health promotion as well as for treatment purpose.

3. Removes obstructions in the channels.

4. Thus allowing the flow of energy throughout the body for revitalizing neergy levels and maintaining equilibrium.

The chart is attatched herewith giving detail areas on the hands and feet, which are linked with internal structures.

Technique

Hold both feet in your hands and establish the contact.

Begin with some rlaxing movements like ankle rotation and ankle stretch.

Stroke the foot softly from ankles to the toes to smooth and

146

relax the whole area of each foot.

Learn techniques like thumb hooking, thumb walking and finger walking.

Find out troubled spots on the sole of the foot.

Select proper oil and massage these points slowly.

3. Shiatsu

Although the roots of this system can be traced to the ancient Chinese medicine like acupuncture, it is modern Japanese therapy. It is a manipulative therapy which uses static pressure applied to specific points and lines all over the body.

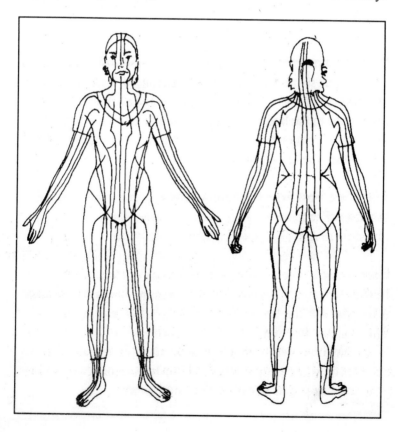

Practioners of this system use their thumbs, elbows, knees and heelsalong the entire netwoek of meridian lines and pressure points. The word 'shi' means finger and 'atsu' means pressure. The main aim of this pressure system on certain points on the body is to prevent diseases and maintain health. This is now recognised in Japan as the traditional system along with the Japanese massage (Asuma).

The important principle of this massage is to have simultaneous touch from both hands. With a two-hand connection, a circuit can be established. Keep one hand stationary, while the other hand moves and can carry out other work.

With the knowledge of the pressure points, Shiatsu expert can diagnose and treat any condition in which there is imbalance in the body energies. Whenever there is any imbalance in the body, toxins accumulate at these points. With the help of proper pressure, one can remove these toxins and bring back the energy balance.

There are 660 zones where vessels, glands, nerves come together. These zones are called as tsubo. Although they are invisible on the skin, experts can locate them.

Hara is one of the most powerful energy centers of the body. In shiatsu terms it is known as the Tanden. The aim of shiatsu is to establish the balance of the body's 'Ki' energy levels. Shiatsu is known to effect claming influences on hypertensions, while people having too low tension can be energized. Many people also find this technique for relieving pain and stress and stress on the mind as well.

<u>Technique</u>
There are two main techniques namely palming and thumbing. In palming place your palms on the body of the patient establish the contact and then exert different pressures on the body.
In other method, the pressure is given by thumbs.

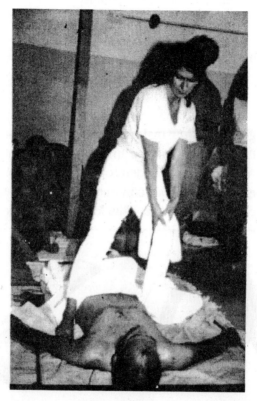

Silk Glove Massage

4. Chiropractic
Daniel David Palmer invented this method of healing. This science belives that most of the physical problems are related

with misaligned or subluxed vertebras and with proper manipulation, they can be well treated. Manipulation used by chiropractors is essentially the same as that of osteopaths, but chiropractors restrict it to the spine, while osteopaths work on joints, even the relatively immobile jonits of cranium.

5. Osteopathy
This is also called as 'bone treatment'. It was invention of Andrew Taylor who was sweedish allopathic doctor.

6. Silk glove massage
Massage with silk gloves is good for kapha constitution persons, as well as for those who have tender skin.

7. Massage with other instruments
At present many electrical instruments having vibratory action as well as other simple wooden rollers are used for massage. They have very limited use compared to the different strokes and medicinal oils and other powders that are used.

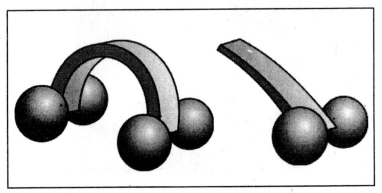

Massage Instruments

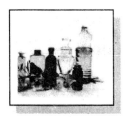

14

Medicated and aromatic oils

Preparation of Medicated oils

Usually 1 part of the kalka or paste of the herbs is mixed with 4 parts of oil and 16 parts of liquid (liquid can be juice of the herbs, decoction or milk etc.) is taken.

First the liquid and the kalka is mixed together then oil is added and the whole mixture is boiled and is stirred continuously, so that the paste does not gets adhered to the bottom of the vessel.

From time to time some paste is taken out of the vessel and its condition is tasted. The medicated oil has three stages of cooking or paka.

1. Mrudu paka - in this stage the paste can be rolled between the fingers

without sticking and is waxy in nature. When kept on fire this wax will burn with slight cracking sound as it contains some amount of water.

2. Madhyama paka- when the mixture is boiled further, the paste becomes

harder and when put into fire, it burns without any cracking noise. The oil prepared upto this stage is used for nasya and for external purpose.

3. Khara paka- when further heat is given to the mixture, the oil has typical

smell and color. At this stage the paste gets fried in the oil. This oil can be used for abhyanga and for basti.

Important Oil Preparations

1. Agaru oil -
Agaru, bilva, yashtimadhu and sesame oil. (BR)

2. Amalaki oil -
Amalaki, haritaki, bibhitaka, bilva, sariva, ela and sesame oil. (BR).

3. Amruta oil -
Tinispora cordifolia, triphala and sesame oil. (BR)

4. Arjuna oil -
Decoction of the bark of arjuna and sesame oil. (YR)

5. Asana eladi oil-
Asana, ela, jeevanti, bilva, bala roots, deodara, sesame oil. (SY).

6. Asana-bilvadi oil-
Asana, bilva, bala, amruta, licorice, triphala, milk, coconut oil. (SY).

7. Ashwagandhadi oil-
Ashwagandha and sesame oil. (BR)

8. Bala oil -
Bala, guduchi, rasna, ela, agaru, manjishtha, atibala, licorice, tulsi, lavanga, kankola, nafgakeshara and sesame oil (AH).

9. Bilvadi oil -
Bilva, goat milk and sesame oil. (SS)

9. Brahmi oil-

Brahmi and coconut oil. (YR)

10. Brihat Saindhavadi oil-
Rock salt (saindhava), arka, maricha, chitraka, haridra and
sesame oil (BR).

11. Bhrungaraja oil -
Eclipta alba, manjishtha, lodhra, bala, daruharidra, licorice,
sandalwood, and sesame oil (BR).

13.Bhrungamalakadi oil-
Juice of bhringaraja and amalaka, licorice, milk and sesame
oil. (SY).

14.Chandanadi oil -
Santalum album, licorice, vetivera zizanoides, jatamansi,
agaru, bala, bilwa, kutki, sesame oil (YR)

15.Chandan-bala-lakshadi oil -
Red and white sandalwood, bala root, laksha, madhuka,
deodaru, manjishtha, agaru, ashwagandha, rasna, katuki, and
sesame oil (YR)

16.Dashamuladi oil-
Dashmula and sesame oil. (YR)

17.Devadarvyadi oil-
Devadaru and sesame oil. (YR)

18.Dhanvantara oil-
Bala roots, cow's milk, kushtha, bilva, patala, agaru,
sandalwood, vacha, punarnava, licorice, sariva, haritaki,
amalaki, (AH and Vaidya Yogaratnavali)

19. Doorvadi oil-
Durva, nimba, narikala ksheera, licorice and coconut oil (AH).

20.Gandha oil -
Herbs in kakolyadi group (kakoli, kshira kakoli, black gram, medha, mahameda, guduchi, jeevanti, kakadshingi, vanshalochana, cow's milk and sesame oil. (AH)

21.Himasagara oil-
Shatavari, kushmanda, vidari, tagara, chandana, manjishtha, agaru, licorice, lodhra, musta, shalmali and sesame oil. (BR)

22.Jeerakadi oil-
Jeeraka and sesame oil. (YR)

23.Jyotishmati oil -
Jyotishmati, apamargaand apamarga. (YR)

24.Karpas-asthyadi oil -
Karpasa seeds, bala, masha, kullatha, sarshapa, rasna, deodaru, punarnava, shigru, kushtha, milk of goat and coconut oil. (SY)

25.Kshara oil -
Plant alkali of apamarga, vacha, shunthi, kushtha, deodaru and sesame oil (BR).

26.Kshirabala oil-
Bala roots, decoction of bala, cow's milk and sesame oil. (AH)

27.Kottamachukadi oil - Kushtha, musta, acorus calamus, garlic, deodaru, sarshapa, curds and sesame oil. (SY)

28.Kumkumadi oil -
Kumkum, ushira, laksha, chandana, yashtimadhu, nagakeshara, manjishtha, teja patra, padmaka, kushtha, gorochana, laksha, daruharidra, priyangu, vacha and sesame oil. (YR)

29.Lakshadi oil -
Laksha, haridra, manjishtha, rasna, ashwagandha and sesame oil. (BR).

30.Lashunadi oil-
Garlic pulp, juice and sesame oil. (CD)

31.Masha oil-
Masha and sesame oil. (BR)

32.Mahamasha oil-
Masha, dashamula, vacha, maricha, gokshura and sesame oil (BR).

33.Mahanarayan oil-
Bilva, ashwagandha, bruhati, gokshura,, bala, kantakari, atibala, rasna, deodaru, agaru, haritaki, ela, licorice, vacha, sesame oil (BR).

34.Manjishthadi oil -
Manjishtha, sariva, musta, katuka, jatiphala, triphala, kushtha, jatamansi, juice of kumari and sesame oil (SY).

35.Maha manjishthadi oil-
Manjishtha, bilva, agnimantha, patala, bruhati, bala, rasna, ashwagandha, punarnava, atibala, sandalwood, manjishtha, kushtha, ela, musta, camphor, sesame oil (BR).

155

36.Nalapamaradi oil -
Juice of fresh curcuma, parpata, udumbara, plaksha, triphala, agaru, kushtha, and sesame oil (SY).

37.Narayan oil -
Shatavari, dashamula, punarnava, ashwagandha, kantakari, jatamansi, vacha, kushtha, milk and sesame oil. (BR)

38.Nimba oil -
Juice of leaves of nimba and sesame oil. (BR)

39.Nimba patradi oil -
Juice of leaves of nimba, eclipta alba, shatavari, manjishtha, licorice, ushira, musta, amruta, sariva, milk and sesame oil (SY).

40.Nirgundi oil (shefali oil) -
Juice of nirgundi and sesame oil.

41.Padmakadi oil-
Lotus stem, doorva, sesame oil. (BR)

42.Pinda oil -
Bee wax, manjishtha, sarjarasa, sariva, dhanyamla, and sesame oil (AH).

43. Sahachara oil -
Sahachara, bilva, gokshura, chandana, shilajita, and sesame oil (AH).

44.Shankhapushpi oil-
Shankhapushpi, bilva, agaru and sesame oil. (YR)

45. Triphaladi oil-
Triphala, guduchi, bala, eranda, kushtha, ushira, musta, milk, sesame oil. (SY)

46. Vacha oil -
Vacha, haritaki, laksha, kutaki and sesame oil. (AH)

47. Vacha lashunadi oil-
Vacha, lashuna and sesame oil. (SY)

48. Vishagarbha oil -
Datura alba, kushtha, vatsanabha, vacha, chitraka and sesame oil (YR).

SEWA PRODUCTS
1. Vata Massage Oil
(Vaidya Yogaratnavali Taila Prakarana)
Use:
Massage for head and body, abhyanga, seka (pouring), nasal drops, enema, vaginal douche. For enema 100 ml of oil should be mixed with 100 ml of boiled milk.
Indication:
For all kinds of vata diseases, especially rheumatic and neurological complaints. Body pain, post-natal care, urinary obstruction, uterine disorders, all orthopedic conditions, pain in the bones, in pregnancy, for children. It will not make disturbances of pitta or kapha. It can be mixed with Kapha Massage Oil, Baby Massage Oil or Sport Massage Oil.

Ingredients:
1. Bala   Sida cordifolia-Indian mallow
2. Water   for decoction
3. Kshira   Milk

4. Yava	Hordeum vulgare-barley
5. Kola	Zizyphus jujuba-Chinese date
6. Kulath	Dolichos biflorus
7. Bilwa	Aegle marmelos
8. Shyonaka	Oroxylum indicum
9. Gambhari	Gmelina arborea
10. Patala	Stereospermum suaveolens
11. Agnimantha	Premna integrifolia
12. Salaparni	Desmodium gangeticum
13. Prsniparni	Pseudarthria viscida
14. Bhrahati	Solanum indicum-Indian bittersweet
15. Kantakari	Solanum virginianum
16. Gokshura	Tribulus terrestris-puncture vine
17. Water	for decoction
18. Taila	Sesamum indicum-sesameoil
19. Meda	Polygonatum cirrihifolium
20. Mahameda	Polygonatum c.-Solomon's seal
21. Daru	Berberis aristata-barberry
22. Manjishta	Rubia cordifolia-madder
23. Kakoli	Lilium polyphyllum-lily
24. Kshirakakoli	Frittillaria roylei
25. Chandana	Santalum album-sandalwood
26. Sariba	Hemidesmus indicus-sarsaparilla
27. Kushta	Saussurea lappa
28. Tagara	Valeriana wallichii
29. Jivakam	Microstylis muscifera
30. Rishabha	Microstylis wallichii
31. Saindhava	Rock salt
32. Kalanusari	Trigonella foenumgraecum
33. Silajit	Slate oil
34. Vacha	Acorus calamus
35. Agaru	Aquillaria agallocha

36. Punarnava   Boerhaavia diffusa
37. Ashwagandha   Withania somnifera
38. Vari   Aspargus racemosus
39. Vidari   Ipomoea mauritiana
40. Yashti   Glycyrrhiza glabra
41. Haritaki   Terminalia chebula
42. Amalaki   Emblica officinalis
43. Bibhitaka   Terminalia belerica
44. Satahva   Peucedanum graveolens
45. Masaparni   Teramnus
46. Mudgaparni   Phaseolus trilobus
47. Ela   Elettaria cardamomum
48. Twak   Cinnamomum zeylanicum
49. Patra   Pogostemon paniculata

2. Pitta Massage Oil
(Asthanga Hridaya, Sutrasthana Chapter 15)
Use:
Massage for head and body, *abhyanga, seka* (pouring).
Indication:
Discoloration of skin, eczema, itching, boils, rhinitis, catarrhal infections, headache, psoriasis (wet type) and skin allergy. Pitta Massage Oil is by nature pitta and kapha reducing. It is effective in skin diseases with itching and blackish discoloration. It will have a more drying effect then sesame oil-based preparations. According to the involvement of pitta of the disease and the constitution of the patient, it can be mixed with ghee.

Ingredients:
1. Ela   Elettaria cardamomum
2. Sukshmela   Heracleum candolleanum
3. Turushka   Vateria indica

4. Kushta   Saussurea lappa
5. Phalini   Callicarpa macrophylla
6. Mamsi   Nardostachys jatamansi
7. Jala   Coleus zeylanicus
8. Spruka   Schizachyrum exile
9. Choraka   Kaempferia galanga
10. Dhyamaka   Schizachyrum exile
11. Patra   Pogostemon paniculata
12. Chocha   Cinnamomum zeylanicum
13. Tagaram   Valeriana wallichi
14. Sthauneya   Taxus baccata
15. Jathi   Myristica fragrans
16. Rasa   Bombax malabarica
17. Sukthi   Calcium of bivalve shells
18. Vyaghranakha-Ipomoea pestigridis
19. Surahva   Cedrus deodara
20. Agaru   Aquillaria agallocha
21. Srivasava   Oinus longifolia
22. Kunkuma   Crocus sativus
23. Chanda Costus speciosus
24. Guggulu   Commiphora mukul
25. Devadhupa   Canarium commune
26. Khapura   Boswellia serrata
27. Punnagum   Calophyllum inophyllum
28. Nagahva   Mesua ferrea
29. Cocunut oil Cocos nucifera
Kapha Massage Oil

(Asthanga Hridaya Cikitsasthana Chapter 21)
Use:
Massage for body, *abhyanga, seka* (pouring), enema. For enema 100 ml of oil should be mixed with 100 ml of boiled milk.

Indication:

3. Kapha Massage Oil

Kapha Massage Oil is more effective in vata diseases affecting the lower limbs like rheumatism, lumbago, sciatica, nervous disorders, varicose veins and vata diseases arising from kapha problems or constitution. Overweight, obesity, weak digestion. It can be mixed with all vata reducing oil. It possesses a slightly heating potency.

Ingredients:

1. Sahachara — Strobilanthus ciliatus
2. Bilwa — Aegle marmelos
3. Syonaka — Oroxylum indicum
4. Gambhari — Gmelina arborea
5. Patala — Stereospermum suaevolens
6. Ganikarika — Premna integrifolia
7. Salaparni — Desmodium gangeticum
8. Prsniparni — Pseudarthria viscida W.& A.
9. Brhati — Solanum indicum
10. Kantakari — Solanum xanthocarpum
11. Gokshura — Tribulus terrestris
12. Shatavari — Asparagus racemosus
13. Usira — Vetiveria zizaniodes
14. Vyaghranakha — Ipomoea pestigridis
15. Kushta — Saussurea lappa
16. Chandana — Santalum album
17. Ela — Elettaria cardamomum
18. Sprukka — Schizachyrum exile
19. Priyangu — Callicarpa macrophylla
20. Nalika — Daemia extensa
21. Hrivera — Coleus zeylanicus
22. Silajit — Slate oil
23. Manjishta — Rubia cordifolia

24. Agaru	Aquilaria agallocha
25. Nalada	Scirpus kysoor
26. Devadaru	Cedrus deodara
27. Kopana	Angelica glauca
28. Misi	Foeniculum vulgaris
29. Turuska	Vateria indica
30. Tagaram	Valeriana wallichii
31. Kshira	Milk
33. Taila	Sesamum indicum

4. Baby Massage Oil

(Asthanga Hridaya)
Use:
Massage for body and head, *abhyanga*, fomentation and enema. For enema 100 ml of oil should be mixed with 100 ml of boiled milk. This is also a very effective cosmetic for the face. Apply the oil at night to the face and you will notify the beautifying and rejuvenating effect on your skin in the morning. In sleeplessness and eye problems it can be applied to the soles of the feet before taking rest.
Indication:
Baby Massage Oil is indicated for vata and vata-pitta diseases, because it will pacify vata without provoking pitta. This is partially due to it's content of milk. It is useful on all types of rheumatic disorders, nervous debility, hypertension, insomnia, rheumatoid arthritis, hemiplegia, facial paralysis. It's tender nutrient nature makes it ideal for baby massage or to strengthen the organism after illness or stress.

Ingredients:
1. Bala juice	Sida cordifolia
2. Bala kalka (paste)	Sida cordifolia

3. Tila	Sesamum indicum
4. Kshira	Cow's milk

5. Sport Massage Oil
(Sahasrayoga Taila Prakarana)
Use:
Massage for body and head, abhyanga, seka (pouring).
Indication:
Effective in Vata-Pitta disorders. Used in rheumatism, rheumatoid arthritis, inflammations, burning sensation, catarrhal conditions and headache.

Ingredients:
1. Bala	Sida cordifolia
2. Guduci	Tinospora cordifolia
3. Devadaru	Cedrus deodara
4. Jatamamsi	Nardostachys jatamansi
5. Kushta	Saussurea lappa
6. Chandana	Santalum album
7. Kundurushka	Boswellia serrata
8. Tagara	Valeriana wallichii
9. Saralam	Pinus roxburghii
10. Rasana	Alpinia galanga
11. Taila	Sesamum indicum

6. Hair Oil

(Sahasrayoga Taila Prakarana)
Use:
Massage for head, shirodhara (pouring on head), shirovasti, gargling, nose drops.
Indication:
Used in loss of hair, graying of hairs, as a hair tonic and to

163

protect from heat, sleeplessness, burning sensation on head, hoarseness of voice, good for eyes and ears, toothache

Ingredients:
1. Bhringaraja   Eclipta alba
2. Amalaka juice   Emblica officinalis
3. Taila   Sesamum indicum
4. Kshira   Cow's milk
5. Madhuka   Madhuca indica

7. Cleansing Powders
General Information
Method of preparation

All ingredients except green and horse gram is collected from the forest properly dried and ground to a very fine powder.

Characteristics

The cleansing powders should bind and neutralize excess oil, sweat, dirt and grease, deep-cleanse the skin or hair without negative drying effect. They possess antiseptic and antiparasitic effects, moisturize the skin and condition the hair. All materials are of vegetable origin. Vetiver is added as natural perfume but acts as well as stimulant and cooling agent and thus prevents prickly heat, itching or inflammations. Neem will not only preserve the powders but serves also as natural anti-septic, anti-viral and insecticide.

Usage

Cleansing powders are a 100 % natural substitute for soaps, shower & bath gels, shampoo's and conditioners.

This can be used even as a peeling or beauty-mask.

They are very useful in pancakarma therapy where oils are used profusely on a daily basis and have to be removed

without disturbing the equilibrium of the skin and hair.
Preservation & Storage

Cleansing Powders should be stored away from heat, light and dampness. If the container is not opened they will preserve safely up to 36 months. After opening the container they should be consumed within six months.

8. Cleansing powder for the skin
Use:

In place of soaps or shower & bath gels, to remove the excess oil after massage or as a peeling if mixed with the following ingredients:

1. with fresh cream or yogurt in vata conditions like dry skin
2. with rose water in pitta conditions like burning sensation, oily skin, eczema etc.
3. with honey in kapha conditions like edema, itching and to promote lymphatic circulation.
4.
Ingredients:
1. Green gram (Phaseolus mungo)
2. Soap berry (Sapindus trifoliatus)
3. Nimba (Azadirachta indica).
4. Horse gram (Dolichos biflorus)
5. Rose petals
6. Pomegranate peel
7. Wild tumeric (Curcuma aromatica)
8. Round zedoary (Curcuma zedoaria)
9. Vetiver

9. Cleansing powder for the hair
Use:

In place of shampoo's and hair conditioners only after

previous application of hair oils, oil massage and other head treatment involving oils.

Ingredients:

1. Shikakayi (Acacia concinna)
2. Soap berry (Sapindus trifoliatus)
3. Nimba (Azadirachta indica)
4. Amla (Emblica officinalis)
5. Green gram (Phaseolus mungo)
6. Rose petals
7. Vetiver

All 'Sewa Ayurveda' products listed above (1to9) are available with Helga M Schmidt, Leutstettener Strasse 67- a. D- 81477 Munchen Germany.

They are also available with 'Vital Force Ayurveda' 9-24 Lloyd Road, Bangalore, 560,009, India.

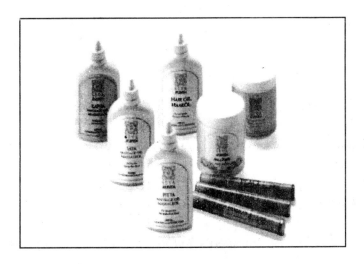

Abbreviations used
AH - Ashtanga hridaya.
BR - Bhaishajya ratnavali.
SS- Siddhayoga Sangraha.
SY - Sahasra yoga.
YR - Yoga ratnakara.

Aromatic Oils
1. Basil - Ocimum sanctum
2. Bay - Pimenta racemosa
3. Benzoin - Stryax benzoin
4. Bergamot - Citrus bergania
5. Cedarwood- Juniperus virginiana
6. Chamomile - Anthemis nobilis
7. Cinnamon - Cinnamomum zeylanicum
8. Comfrey - Symphtum offiicnale
9. Cypress - Cupressus sempervirens
10. Eucalyptus - Eucalyptus globulus
11. Fennel- Foeniculum vulgare
12. Frankincense- Boswellia thurifera
13. Geranium- Pelargonium adorantissimum
14. Hyssop- Hyssopus officinalis
15. Jasmine - Jasminum officinale
16. Juniper- Juniperus communis
17. Lavender - Lavendula officinalis
18. Lemon - Citrus limonum
19. Lemongrass- Cymbopogon citratus
20. Marjoram - Origanum marjorana
21. Melissa - Melisa officinalis
22. Myrrh- Comiphora myrrh
23. Neroli- Citrus aurantium
24. Orange- Citrus aurantium or sinesis

25. Parsley -Petroselinum sativum
26. Patchouli- Pogostemon patchouli
27. Peppermint- Mentha piperata
28. Pine- Pinus sylvestris
29. Rose- Rosa centigolia
30. Rosemary - Rosamarinus officinalis
31. Sage- Salvia officinalis
32. Sandalwood - Santalum album
33. Tea Tree- Melaleuca alternifolia
34. Thyme- Thymus vulgaris
35. Ylang -Ylang- Cananga odorata

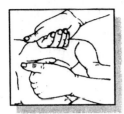

15.
Research on Massage

All over the world, various medical Institutes has done research on the effects of massage, their relations with the physiology of the body as well as the effect of massage in different diseases.

The Medical Library at Bethesda, USA; has collected this research data. Now this research is available in India with National Informatic Center, Pune in 'Medlars and Gistnic Database' section. The information available with this section is really vast as it contains more than 600 pages. We have only given some important research work in this chapter.

1. Stress and Strain
Effects of brief massage therapy, music relaxation with visual imagery on muscle relaxation at a major public hospital. The effects were assessed using a within subjects pre-post test design in 100 emplyoes. Result showed that the therapies, when applied for short periods of time, are equally effective for reducing stress among hospital employees. University of Miami School of Medicine, Florida, 33101, USA
2. Aromatherapy and massage for geriatric care
The appropriate use of these therapies is useful in convential treatment regimens. Associate degree Nursing program, Ohio University of Zenesville, USA

3. Headache

Footreflex zone massage was found effective. Institute fur Pflegeforschung, Bern, Germany.

4. Use of massage in Sports medicine

Massage is beneficial to increase blood flow, healing of connective tissues and edema. School of ocupational therapy and Physiotherapy, University of east Angelia, Norwich, UK.

5. Peptic ulcer and GI tract diseases

Compared to conventional treatment, deep reflex muscular massage for treatment of peptic ulcer patients show positive changes in adaptive compensatory systems.

6. Tension headaches

81 patients were treated with massage, vibration etc. Excellent results were obtained. JFK medical center, Wellington regional medical center, Atlantis, Florida, USA.

7. Pressure sores

Regular massage of the bony prominance can prevent bedsores. Maastritcht Uniersity, Faculty of health sciences, Department of Nursing science, Nedarlands.

8. Cerebral circulatory disorders

119 patinets who have suffered an episode of reversible brain ischaemia were studid in this project. To find out the effect of massage of different areas of the body on the cerebral hemodynamics.

9. Job stress

Short massage therapy produced immediate relief in persons working in hospital. University of Miami, USA.

10. Asthma

32 children with asthma were randomly assigned to receive massage or relaxation therapy. The younger children who received massage showed immediate decrease in behavioural anxiety and improved pulmonary functions. Touch Research Institute, University of Miami, USA.

11. Chronic low backache

Relaxation, corrective manual modulation and improving postural drawbacks produced great relief. Christie clinic association, Dept. of Sports Medicine, Rantoul, IL, 61866 USA

12. Cancer pain

Development of massage service to cancer patients as complimentary therapy is useful in reducing many problems. Radiotherapy department, Hammersmith hospital, London, UK. And Northwestern Ontario Regional Cancer Center. Canada

13. Pregnancy

26 pregnant women were assigned to massage therapy for 5 weeks. This produced reduction in anxiety, improved mood, better sleep and less back pain. Touch Research Institute, Florida, USA.

14. Sleep disturbance

Critically ill patients are deprived of sleep and its healing qualities. 69 patients were randomly selected and were given 6 minute back massage along with 6-minute relaxation technique. It was found out that back massage was useful for promoting sleep. University of Arkansas, College of nursing, Little rock, USA.

15. Postmastectomy lymphoedema and massage

Multimodel therapy reduced lymphadematous limb volume by atleast in 18 out of 25 patients. Wesley Clinic for haematology and Oncology.

16. Chromassi

is a system based on Chrono-massage, which is used for painful syndromes and chronic diseases. This is a combination of massage and acupressure. The system can be used for teaching and clinics. This can be run on PC computers.

Institute of computer science, Academy of sciences, Prague, Czech Republic.

16.
Index of Botanical Herbs

SANSKRIT	ENGLISH	BOTANICAL
Abhaya	Myrobalan	Terminalia chebula
Agaru	Eaglewood	Aquilaria agallocha
Agasti	Agati	Sesbania grandiflora
Agnimantha	Clerodendrum	phlomidis
Agnimantha		Premna integrifolia
Ahiphena	Opium	Papaver somniferum
Ajagandha	-	Gynandropsis pentaphylla
Ajamoda	Cellary seed	Carum ajmoda / roxburghianum
Akarakarabha	Pellitory roots	Anacyclus pyrethrum
Akshotaka	Wall Nut	Juglans regia
Amalaki	Embellic myrobalans	emblica/ officinalis
Amaravel	Doddar	Cuscuta reflaxa
Amlavetasa	-	Garcinia pedunculata
Amlavetasa	Sorrel	Rumex vesicarius
Amra	Mango	Magnifera indica
Amragandhi haridra	-	Curcuma amada
Amruta	-	Tinospora cordifolia

Ananta	Indian sarsaparela	Hemidesmus indicus
Apamarga	Rough chapp tree	Achyranthes aspera
Aparajita	Butterfly pea	Clitoria ternatea
Aragvadha		Casia fistula
Arishtaka trifoliatus	Soap nut	Sapindus
Arjuna	Arjuna Myrobalan	Terminalia arjuna
Arka	Calotropis	Calotropis procera
Asana	-	Pterocarpus marsupium
Ashoka	Ashok Tree	Saraca indica
Ashvagol	-	Plantago ovata
Ashwagandha	Winter cherry	Withania somnifera
Ashwattha	-	Ficus religiosa
Asthisandhanaka	-	Cissus quadrangularis
Atasi	Linseed	Linum usitatissimum
Atibala	Indian Mellow	Abutilon indicum
Ativisha	Indian Attees	Aconitum heterophyllum
Avartaki	Tanners Cassia	Cassia auriculata
Avartani	Indian Screwtree	Helicteres isora
Babbula	Indian Gum Tree	Acacia
Bakuchi	Bavachi	Psoralea corylifolia
Bakula	Indian Medler	Mimusops elengi
Bala	-	Sida cordifolia
Banapsha	-	Viola odorata
Bhallataka	Marking Nut	Semicarpus

		anacardium
Bhanga		Cannabis sativa
Bharangi	-	Clerodendrum indicum
Bhringaraja	-	Eclipta alba
Bibhitaka		Terminalia chebula
Bilva	Bael	Aegle marmelos
Bola	-	Commiphora myrrh
Brahmi	Indian Pennywort	Bacopa moniera
Bruhati	Indian Nightshade	Solanum indicum
Chakramarda	Foetid cassia	Cassia tora
Champaka	-	Michelia champaka
Chandana	Sandalwood	Santalum album
Chandrashura	Watercress	Lepidium sativum
Changeri	-	Oxalis corniculata
Chavika / Chavya	-	Piper chaba
Chincha		Tamarindus indica
Chitrak rakta	Leadwort	Plumbago rosea
Chitraka	Leadwort	Plumbago zeylanica
Chopachini	China root	Smilax china
Dadima	Pomegranate	Punica granatum
Danti	-	Baliospermum mortanum
Danti	Wild croton	Croton polyandrum
Daruharidra	Indian barberies	Barberis aristata
Davana	-	Artemissia palenf
Devdaru	Doddar	Cedrus deodara
Dhanyaka	Coriander	Coriandrum

175

		sativum
Dhataki	Fulsee flower	Woodfordia fruticosa
Dhatriphala	-	Barringtonia acutangula
Dhatura Krishna	Thorn apple	Datura metal
Dhatura shweta	Thorn apple	Datura stramonium
Draksha	Grape	Vitis vinifera
Dronapushpi	-	Leucas cephalotes
Duralabha /Dhanvayasa	-	Fagonia cretica Alhagi pseudalhagi
Durva	Creeping cyndon	Cyndon dactylon
Ela	Lesser cadamum	Elettaria cardamomum
Erandkarkati	Papaya tree	Carica papaya
Erandmool	Castor oil tree	Ricinus communis
Falgu	Fig Tree	Ficus carica
Gajapippali	Elephant piper	Scindapsus officinalis
Gambhari	White teak	Gmelina arborea
Gandha shathi	-	Hedychium spicatum
Gangeruki	-	Canthium parviflorum
Garjar	Carrot	Daucus carota
Gojivha	-	Onosma bracteatum
Gokshura	Calitrops	Tribulus terrestris
Guduchi	-	Tinospora cordifolia
Guggul	-	Balsamodendron mukul
Gunja	Bead Tree	Abrus precatorius

Hamspadi	Maidan hair	Adiantum lunulatum
Hapuspha	Junipar	Juniperus communis
Haridra	Turmeric	Curcuma longa
Hasishudha		Heliotropium indicum
Hingu	Assafoetida	Ferula assafoetida
Hingupatri	White emetic nut	Peucedanum grande
Hriber		Pavonia deodorata
Ikshu	Sugarcane	Saccharum officinarum
Indravaruni	Colocynth, apple	Citrullus bitter colocynthis
Indrayawa	Kurchi	Holerrhena antidysenterica
Ingudi	Zacum oil plant	Balanites ingudi
Irimeda	-	Acacia farnesiana / leucopholea
Isabgol	Spogel	Plantago ovata
Ishvari	Indian birchwort	Aristolchia indica
Jaiphala	Croton seed	Croton tiglium
Jambira	Lemon	Citrus medica
Jambu	Black plum	Eugenia jambolana
Jatamasi jatamasi	Musk root	Nardostachys
Jatipatri	/Mace	Myristica fragrans
Jatiphal	Nutmeg	Myristica fragrans
Jiraka	Cumin seed	Cuminum cyminum
Jivanti	-	Leptadenia reticulata

177

Jyotishmati paniculatus	Stuff tree.	Celastrus
Kababchini	Cubeb	Piper cubeba
Kadamba	Cadamba	Anthocephalus cadamba
Kadli	Banana	Musa sapientum / paradisiaca
Kakajangha	-	Leea acquata
Kakmachi	Black night shade	Solanum nigrum
Kakmari	-	Anamirta cocculus
Kalmegh	Creat	Andrographis paniculata
Kampilla	Kamilla	Mallotus philippinensis
Kanchanara	-	Bauhinia variegata
Kandiari	Jujube fruit	Zinziphus mauritiana/ phillippinesis
Kantakari	-	Solanum xanthocarpum
Kapikachchu	Cowhage plant	Mucuna pruriens
Kapittha	Wood apple	Feronia elephantum
Karanja	Beach	Pongomia glabra
Karchura	-	Hedychium spicatum
Karkatashringhi	Galls	Rhus succedanea
Karpas	Indian cotton	Gossypium herbaceum
Karpura	Camphor	Cinnamomum camphora
Karvira	-	Nerium indicum
Kasani		Cicorum endiva

Kasmarda	Round poded cassia	Cassia occidentalis
Katphala	Box myrtal	Myrica nagi
Katuka	Hellbore	Picrorhiza kurroa
Ketaki	Keora	Pandanus odoratissim
Khadira	Catechu tree	Acacia catechu
Kharjura	Date palm	Phoenix dactylifera
Kirata	Chiretta	Swertia chirata
Kirmani	-	Artemisia maritima
Kitmari yavani	-	Aristolchia bracteata
Kokilaksha	-	Asteracantha longifolia
Krushna jiraka	Caroway seeds	Carum carvi
Kuberaksha	Bondu	Caesalpinia bonducella
Kulattha	-	Dolichos biflorus
Kulinjana	Galangal	Alpinia officinarum
Kumari	Aloes	Aloe vera
Kumuda	-	Nymphaea alba
Kunkuma	Saffron	Crocus sativus
Kupilu	-	Strychnus nuxvomica
Kushmanda	-	Benincasa hispida
Kushtha	Costus	Sausurea lappa
Kutaj	Conessi bark	Holarrhena antidysenteria
Lajjalu	Sensitive plant	Mimosa pudica
Laksha	Lac	Cocculus lack
Langali	Superbily	Gloriosa superba

Lashuna	Garlic	Allium sativum
Latakaranja	-	Caesalpinia crista
Lavanga	Clove	Syzygium aromatica
Lodhra	Lodhra	Symplocos recemosa
Lohban	-	Styrax benzoin
Madana	Emetic nut	Randia dumetorum
Madayantika	-	Lawsonia inermis
Madhuka	Mahua tree	Bassia latifolia
Mahanimba	-	Melia azadirachta
Maiphala	-	Quercus infectoria
Majuphala	Gallnut	Quercus infectoria
Mamira	-	Coptis teeta
Mandukaparni	-	Hydrocotyl asiatica
Manjatak	-	Eulophia compestris
Manjistha	Madder root	Rubia cordifolia
Mansala	Guava	Psidium guyava
Maricha (rakta)	Red chili	Capsicum fruitescens
Maricha	Black pepper	Piper nigrum
Markandi	Senna	Cassia angustifolia
Mashaparni	-	Termanus labialis
Matulunga	Adams apple	Citrus medica
Mendika	Henna	Lawsonia alba
Methika	Fenugreek	Trigonella foenum-graceum
Mnjatak	Salep	Eulophia compestris
Mocharas	-	Bombax malabaricum
Moolaka	Garden radish	Raphanus sativus

Moorva	-	Clematis triloba
Muchkunda	-	Pterospermum indicus
Mudga		Phaseolus radiatus
Mundi	-	Sphaeranthus indicus
Musli (black)	-	Curculigo orchioides
Musli	-	Asparagus adscendens
Musta	Nutgrass	Cyeperus rotundus
Nadihingu	Gummy gardenia	Gardenia gummifera
Nagarjuni	Australian asthama weed	Euphorbia pilulifera
Nagkeshar	Cobras Saffron	Mesua ferrea
Narikel	Coconut	Cocos nucifera
Nilika	Indigo	Indigofera tinctoria
Nimbuka	Lemon	Citrus acida
Nirgundi	-	Vitex negundo
Nirvishi	-	Delphinium denudatum
Padma	Lotus	Nelumbium speciosum
Padmaka	Himalayan cherry	Prunus cerasoides
Palandu	Onion	Allium cepa
Palash	Butta	Butea frondosa
Parasika yavani	-	Hyocymus reticulata
Parasika Yavani	Henbane	Hyocymus niger
Paribhadra	Indian coral tree	Erythrina indica
Parijataka	-	Nyctanthus arborstristis

Parnabeeja	-	Kalanchoe pinneta
Pashanabheda	-	Bergenia ligulata
Patanga	Sappan wood	Cacsesalpinia sapan
Patla	Trumpet flower Guard	Stereospermum suaveslens
Patola	Wild Snake	Trichosanthes dioica
Pippala	Sacred Fig	Ficus religiosa
Pippali	Long Pepper	Piper longum
Pippalimoola	-	Piper longum roots
Pishach Karpas	Abrona	Abroma augusta
Pitta Papara	-	Fumaria officinalis
Priyala	-	Buchanania latifolia
Priyalaka	-	Buchanania latifolia
Priyangu	Aglaia roxburghiana	Callicarpa macrophylla
Prushniparni	-	Uraria logopoides
Pruthvika	-	Nigella sativa
Puga	Betel nut	Areca catechu
Punarnva rakta	Spreading hogwood	Boerhaavia diffusa
Pushkaramula	-	Inula racemosa
Putiha	-	Mentha spicata
Putrajivaka	-	Putranjiva roxburghi
Rakta chandan	Red sandal	Pterocarpus santalinus
Rakta niryas	Indian kino tree	Calamus draco
Rasanjana	Barberis	Berberis aristata
Rasna	-	Vanda roxburghii

182

Revand chini	-	Rheum emodi
Rohitak	-	Ammora rohitak
Rudraksha	-	Elaeocarpus ganitrus
Sahachar	Yellow nadar	Barleria prionitis
Sahadevi	-	Vernonia cinerea
Samudra Palak	Elephant creeper	Argyreia speciosa
Saptaparni	Dita	Alstonia scholaris
Saptarangi	-	Caeseria esculanta
Sarala	Longleave pine	Pinus longifolia / roxburghi
Sariva	-	Hemidesmus indicus
Sarja	-	Vateria indica
Sarpagandha	-	Rauwolfia serpentina
Shal	Yellow resin	Shorea robusta
Shalaparni	Ticktrefoil	Desmodium gangeticum
Shalmali	-	Bombax malabaricum
Shankhapushpi	-	Convolvulus microphyllus
Sharpunkha	Purple tephrosia	Tephrosia purpurea
Shatavari	Asparagus	Asparagus racemosus
Shatavha	Dill	Peucedanum graveolens
Shati	Zeodary	Curcuma zedoaria
Shatpushpa	Fennel	Foeniculum vulgare
Shigru /Shobhanjana	Drumstick tree	Moringa pterygosperma

Shirish	-	Albizzia lebbeck
Shunthi	Ginger root	Zingiber officinalis
Shwet Dhatura	-	Datura alba
Shwet Kanchan	Common mountain ebony	Bauhinia recemosa
Shyonaka		Oroxylum indicum
Snuhi	-	Euphorbia nerifolia
Somlata	Ephedra	Epherdra vulgaris
Sudarshan	-	Crinum zeylanicum
Suran	-	Amorphophalus companullatus
Surinjan	Colchicum	Colchicum luteum
Suvarnaka	Indian labournam	Cassia fistula
Suvarnakshiri	Yellow thistle	Argemone mexicana
Tagara	Indian valerian	Valeriana wallichii
Talispatra	-	Abies webbina
Tamal Patra	Tamala	Cinnamomum tamala
Tambula	Betel leaf	Piper betel
Tila	Sesame	Sesamum indicum
Tinduka	Ebony	Diospyros embryopteris
Tintidika	Tamarind	Tamarindus indica
Trayanti	Gold thread	Delphinium zalil
Trivruta	Turpeth root	Ipomea turpethum
Tulsi	Basil	Ocimum sanctum
Tuveraka	Chalmogra	Hydnocarpus wightiana
Twak	Cinnamon	Cinnamomum zeylanicum

Udumbara	Fig tree	Ficus glomerata
Ushira	Cuscus grass	Vetiveria zizaniodes
Vacha	Sweet flag	Acorus calmus
Vanharidra	Wild turmeric	Curcuma aromatica
Vanshlochana	Bamboo camphor	Bamboo manna
Varuna	-	Crataeva religiosa
Vasaka	Vasaka	Adhatoda vasica
Vata	Banyan Tree	Ficus bengalensis
Vatasnabha	Aconite	Aconitum ferox
Vatghani	Wind killer	Clerodendeum phlomidis
Vidanga	Vidanga	Embelia ribes
Vidari	-	Pueraria taberosa
Vijaya	Indian hemp	Cannabis indica
Vijayasara	Indian kino tree	Pterocarpus marsupium
Vishatinduka	Nux vomica	Strychnos nuxvomica
Yashtimadhu	Liquorice	Glycerrhiza glabra
Yava	Barly	Hordeum valgare
Yavasaka	Comb thorn	Alhagi camelorum
Yawani	Bishopweed	Carum copticum

17.
Sanskrit English Glossary

Abhighata sahatva- increases imunity to bear trauma
Abhyanga - application of oil to the body
Adhipati - the overlord
Aghata- percussion
Alochaka - sub-type of Pitta, for subtle digestion required for sense organs
Ama -toxin
Amsa - shoulder
Anguli peedana- kneading with cushion of fingers
Anuloma - in the direction of hairs
Apana- sub-type of Vata, controlling downward movement of feces, urine etc
Asthi- bone
Asthigata Vata- osteo arthritis
Atharva Veda- type of Veda
Avalambaka -sub- type of kapha, protecting lungs
Avapeedana- light kneading
Ayu - life
Ayu kara- promotes longevity
Ayurveda - Science of life
Basti- bladder
Bhrajaka - sub-type of Pitta, digestion of oils and medicines applied to skin
Bodhaka -sub- type of kapha, protecting buccal cavity
Brahmrandra - anterior fontenale
Chavitti - massage with feet
Chedyam- hacking
Dhatu - tissue

Dosha - biological humor
Droni- Traditional wooden table for massage
Drushti prasada kara- beneficial to eyes
Dugdha dhara - drip of milk on head
Gharshana - to rub
Guda- anus
Gulpha - ankle joint
Harshana- vibration
Hridaya- heart
Janu- knee joint
Kampa - vibration
Karna purana- filling the ears with oil
Kesamardana- shampooing the hairs
Kleda - subtle waste product
Kleda - Subtle waste product.
Kledaka - sub-type of kapha, protecting G I tract
Klesha sahatva- increases strength of the skin to bear pain
Kshipra - quick
Kundalini - serpant power lying dormant at the base of the spine.
Kurcha- knot or bundle of muscles
Lata-veshtana- spiral friction
Mahabharata- Mythological epic
Mala - waste product
Mamsa- facia
Mandhana- muscle rolling
Mardana- massage with pressure
Marma - vital point
Meda - fatty tissue
Mohan-jo-daro - ancient city at the time of Veda
Nabhi- naval
Nasya- nasal medication

Navarakizi - massage with rice bolus
Netra basti - bathing eye in ghee or oil
Netra tarpana- bathing eye with ghee or oil
Nirama - without toxin
Pachaka - sub-type of Pitta, for primary digestion of the food
Padaghata - massage with feet
Pari-peedana- Petrissage
Peedana - kneading
Phenaka - producing lather foam
Pichu - cotton swab
Pichu dharana - holding or keeping cotton dipped in oil on head
Pizichil - massage with warm oil drip
Praharana- percussion
Prakruti - bio-typology, constitution
Prana - sub-type of Vata, controlling inward movement of food, air, water
Pra-peedana- deep kneading
Pratiloma - opposite to the direction of hairs
Pushtikara - nourishes body
Rakta - particulate matter in the blood
Ramayana- Indian mythological epic
Ranjaka - sub-type of Pitta, for secondary digestion
Rasa- plasma
Sadhaka - sub-type of Pitta, for digestion of knowledge
Sama - with ama
Samana- sub- type of Vata, controlling movement of all hormones and digestive juices in G I tract
Sama-prakruti- balanced constitution
Samvahana - massage
Sandhi-chalana- movement of joints
Sandhigata Vata- rheumatoid arthritis
Seemanta- the summit, the scull and surrounding joints

Shikha- crest of the skull
Shiro dhara- (oil) drip on the head
Shiro mardana- head massage
Shleshaka - sub-type of kapha, protecting joints
Shrama hara- removes fatigue
Shrungataka- place where four roads meet
Shukra- reproductive tissue
Snayu - muscle
Snehana -oleation, lubrication
Sparsha- touch
Sthapani- what gives support
Sutwak kara- makes skin soft
Swapna kara- gives proper sleep
Swedana - fomentation
Takra dhara - drip of buttermilk on head
Talahridaya - heart of the palm and sole
Tarpaka - sub-type of kapha, protecting brain
Trasana - stroking
Udana - sub-type of Vata, controlling outward movement of air
Udgharshana - reinforced friction
Udvartana- massage with dry powders
Udveshtana- wringing
Utsadana - massage with herbal paste
Uzichil- massage with medicated herbs
Vaadyam- tapping
Vatarakta- gouty arthritis
Veda - knowledge
Vitap - perinium
Vyana - sub-type of Vata, controlling movements of heart, muscles

18.
Bibliography

1. Ashtang hridaya
2. Better health with foot Reflexology - Dwight Byers.
3. Bhavaprakasha
4. Charaka samhita
5. Encyclopedia of aromatherapy Massage and Yoga- Carole Mcgilvery, Jim Reed, Mira Mehta. Smith Mark Publishers, New York, USA
6. Gentle art of healing - Dr. Hans H. Rhyner
7. Health and Healing- Andrew Weil, Houghton Mifflin Company, Boston, USA
8. Indian ancient massage- Harish Johari
9. Mardanashatra - Vaidya M.P.Nanal, Dr. R.K. Garde
10. Massage - Stewart Mitchell
11. Massage at your fingertips - Science of life books, Melbourne, Australia.
12. Massage therapy in Ayurveda - Vaidya Bhagavan Dash, Concept publishing company, New Delhi.
13. Natural health,Natural medicine- Andrew Weil, Houghton Mifflin Company, Boston, USA
14. Panchakarma and Ayurvedic Massage -by Dr. Lele, Dr. Subhash Ranade and Dr. Qutab Published by International Academy of Ayurveda, Erandavana, Pune 411,004).
15. River of Heven - Dr. David Frawley
16. Sushruta samhita
17. Vatsyaya kamasutra, (yashodhara commentary)
18. Yogratnakara

Resources

Diploma courses on massage are conducted at the following centers :-

1. Ateneo Veda Vyasa
Yoga Sadhana Ashram, 17041, Altare, Savona, Italy
Tel/Fax - 0039-19-584838
E mail - ashram@tnt.it
Offers one year Ayurveda course.

2. Ayurveda Clinic
Rajbharati, 367 Sahakar Nagar1,Pune 411 009,
Director- Dr. Sunanda Ranade
Tel/Fax 0091-20-4224427
E mail - snranade@hotmail.com
Offers Ayurvedic Counselling.

3. Ayurvedic Institute of America.
Walnut Grove Lane, Coppel, Texas, 75019, U.S.A.
Tel. 001-972-462-1919
E mail - jayapte@aol.com
Director, Dr. Jay Apte
Offers one year Ayurveda Course.

4. Ayurvedic Acupuncture Board of Acreditation
19, Bowy Avenue, Enfield, SA, 5085, Australia.
Director - Dr. Frank Ros
Tel./Fax 0061-08-83497303
E mail - suchi-Karma@picknow.com au

5. California College of Ayurveda

135 Argyl Way, Suit B, Nevada City, CA, 95959, U.S.A.
Tel.001-530-274-9100
E mail - CCA@oro.net
Director - Dr. Marc Halpern
Offers 18 months Ayurveda Course.

6. East West College of Herbalism

Hartswood, Marshgreen, Hartsfoeld, Sussex TN7 4ET,U.K.
Tel.0044-1342-822312
E mail - EWCOLHERB@aol.com
Director- David and Sarah Holland
Offers 3 years Diploma course of Ayurveda.

7. Foundation for Health Promotion - Fundacja Pomocy Zdrowiu

Ul.Belletiego 1, 01-022 Warsaw, Poland
Tel. 0048-22-6363401
Director-Zanna Kiesner
E mail - hacenter@kki.net.pl

8. International Academy of Ayurveda

Atrey Rugnalaya and Research Institute, M.Y.Lele Chowk,
Erandawana, Pune 411 004, India.
Tel/Fax -0091-20-5678532
Director-Dr. Avinash Lele.
E mail - avilele@hotmail.com
Offers basic and advance Ayurveda Training, Panchakarma and counselling.
Website: http://www.ayurved-int.com

9. Janaki Clinic and Panchakarma Health Spa

Karvenagar, Pune - 411052, India.